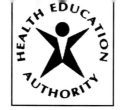

CW00815874

Drug Education and Prevention Handbook

A 'snapshot' of organisations and activities

ACKNOWLEDGEMENTS

The Health Education Authority wishes to thank all the organisations, projects and agencies which have been included for their co-operation and assistance during the production of this handbook.

Our special thanks are extended to Sarah Waterton, Steve Taylor and Elspeth Sutherland of the Standing Conference on Drug Abuse for their inexhaustible commitment and enthusiasm; thanks also to Victoria Fitch (consultant to the HEA), Liz Niman (HEA editor), Stuart Watson (Senior Project Manager, HEA Drugs Programme).

This work was funded by the Department of Health as part of the drugs strategy for England, *Tackling Drugs Together* (HMSO, 1995).

This handbook contains information on drug education and prevention which should be useful to Drug Action Teams, Drug Reference Groups, local drug service staff and other health professionals. It represents one element of a much larger HEA drugs campaign. For more information on the drugs work of the HEA, see page 44.

Health Education Authority
Trevelyan House
30 Great Peter Street
London SW1P 2HW

Typeset by Type Generation Ltd, London EC1
Printed in Great Britain by The Cromwell Press

ISBN 0 7521 0713 5

Contents

Overview

The Health Education Authority (HEA) was commissioned by the Department of Health in May 1995 to run a three-year publicity and information campaign to highlight the health risks associated with the use of illicit drugs and solvent abuse. This campaign forms part of the wider government strategy for England, *Tackling Drugs Together* (HMSO, 1995) which works across several government departments and covers all aspects of illicit drug use.

It has long been recognised that there is no single approach to effective drug education and prevention, and the work is the domain of no single agency – intervention involves a variety of organisations employing a range of techniques. However, the potential for a national initiative linked to local action on drugs is immense, with the greatest impact likely to be achieved through a national programme in combination with local activities. For such an approach to be successful, all agencies involved in drug education and prevention (from the purchasers and providers of prevention activity to Drug Action Teams, and non-drug specialist professionals and agencies) must be able to access both locally and nationally, the relevant skills, expertise, and other related services and networks, to allow the exchange of information and ideas to take place.

To facilitate this process, in 1996, the HEA commissioned the Standing Conference on Drug Abuse (SCODA) to develop a database of a range of agencies involved in drug education and prevention work in England. This handbook is based on the information contained in that database.

In chapter 1, the background to drug education and prevention work is outlined, and the methods and criteria used for data collection are then detailed in chapter 2. Examples of local project work are included in chapter 3 to give the handbook a sense of reality and practice. Local activities are presented in the Directory section of the handbook – in order to maximise accessibility organisations and activities are listed by geographical location (page 315), by Drug Action Team area (page 323) and organisations are also listed alphabetically (page 330). Information on other local services is in chapter 4, and national organisations in chapter 5. There are also appendices providing basic guidance on sources of funding and on related literature.

This handbook is designed to enable readers to find out:

● what kinds of activities and projects are being run at local level, which groups they are targeting and which methods they are using, and to provide contact information for those activities;

- how particular activities managed to put their aims and objectives into practice;
- how local and district services are involved;
- which national organisation to contact with a specific enquiry.

There are a wide range of organisations and activities involved in drug education and prevention. It was recognised at the outset that this first mapping project and handbook could only provide a 'snapshot of a field in motion'. During the production of this handbook, we were aware that due to the short-term nature of many activities, some of those listed in the Directory were no longer running or about to be completed. These activities are included to demonstrate the range of work taking place and to give an overview of the field.

The information contained within the handbook is correct to the best of our knowledge at the time of writing. The information in the Directory section was provided by the local organisations and activities through self-completion questionnaires (see Appendix 3 for a sample questionnaire). The inclusion of examples of local activities does not imply any form of endorsement. Exclusion of a particular organisation or activity in no way implies that its work is not of a high standard.

Organisations included in the Directory are willing to provide further information about their work; therefore contact details have been included.

Since the completion of this handbook, the HEA has commissioned SCODA to pilot LOCATE, a Drug Education and Prevention Information Service to extend both the scope of the original database and to provide a direct service to people working in the drugs field including local drug service staff and other health professionals. Requests for information should be forwarded to LOCATE, Drug Education and Prevention Information Service, SCODA, 32–36 Loman Street, London SE1 0EE, Tel: 0171-803 4733, Fax: 0171-928 3343. The pilot will run initially until March 1998.

It is intended that the handbook will be updated. We welcome your comments on the development of this ongoing project. Please send your comments to SCODA, 32–36 Loman Street, London SE1 0EE.

Hannah Cinamon
Programme Manager
Drugs Programme
Health Education Authority

Joan Heuston
Senior Research Manager
Drugs Programme
Health Education Authority

Chapter 1

Drug education and prevention activities: background and current situation

Introduction

The national drug strategy for England is set out in *Tackling Drugs Together* (1995). A major focus of this strategy is to discourage young people from taking drugs and for those unable or unwilling to stop using drugs, to minimise the harm or risks involved in drug use both to individuals and to communities.

The Advisory Council on the Misuse of Drugs (ACMD) defined preventative measures as having to satisfy two basic criteria:

- to reduce the risk of an individual engaging in drug misuse;
- to reduce the harm associated with drug misuse (Home Office, 1984).

More recently, the Health Advisory Service review (HAS, 1996) adopted the following definitions.

According to the review, education is not training:

> 'Training refers to the education of the staff of services whereas…education of children and adolescents…about substances has the overall aim of preventing people from harming themselves by the use of substances.'

The term 'prevention' by contrast, is defined as embracing:

> 'the promotion of lower risk use or harm-minimisation. This includes prevention of dependent forms of substance misuse and prevention of physical and psychiatric disorders that may be related to substance use and misuse.'

Factors affecting drug education and prevention activities

Drug education and prevention encompass many different kinds of work involving and targeting children, young people and adults. However, there is no consistent understanding of the most appropriate way to deliver effective messages or the overall approach that should be taken. Complex and interrelated factors influence the decisions made by agencies regarding the aim, content and method of their programmes. Some of these factors are looked at below.

Interpretation of 'drug education' and 'drug prevention'

The philosophy and values of an agency, its function and the definitions it uses affect the services it offers. Agencies often have a specific interpretation of drug education and prevention in mind when delivering their programmes, although this is not always made explicit. The two terms 'drug education' and 'drug prevention' are adopted either separately or in combination, but are often used loosely and interchangeably.

Agency specialisation

Approaches to drug education and prevention may concentrate on one or other of the aims of education and prevention. This makes for a wide spectrum of initiatives, from those which accept that many young people are likely to have experience of some drug use, to those which anticipate no drug use (abstinence) as being the starting and finishing point of their education.

Type of agency

A wide range of agencies and professionals are involved in drug education and prevention, including:

- health sector (GPs, nurses, health visitors, health promotion officers);
- social services (social workers and care managers);
- education (schools and colleges);
- law enforcement, criminal justice and community safety organisations (police, probation officers, local authority planning and/or environment employees);
- specialist drug services;
- statutory and voluntary youth services;
- arts and sports organisations.

These agencies and professionals often work in partnership, and many take a holistic approach to individual or group work with young people. This means that agencies incorporate drug education and prevention work into their broader brief to influence young people's behaviour and attitudes towards their health, education or welfare.

Target group

The age, experience of drugs, background, motivations, ethnicity, culture and size of the target group are just some of the factors which determine the type of drug education and the prevention messages that may be appropriate. For example, young people may respond better to drug education which is provided by their peers rather than by their parents; younger children are less likely to be involved in any form of illegal drug use and education will often start from the basis of parental use of medicines and alcohol; drug education with 17-year-old rave goers would need to take into account that drug use may already be an intrinsic part of the experience of the target group.

Settings

In school

Official guidelines on drug education and prevention in schools were set out in the Department for Education circular *Drug prevention and schools* (DfE, 1995). This refers to the revised National Curriculum Science Order for England and Wales, which states that pupils should be taught:

- at Key Stage 1 (5–7-year-olds) about the role of drugs as medicines;
- at Key Stage 2 (7–11-year-olds) that tobacco, alcohol and other drugs can have harmful effects;
- at Key Stage 3 (11–14-year-olds) that the abuse of alcohol, solvents, tobacco and other drugs affects health, that the body's natural defence may be enhanced by immunisation and medicines; and how smoking affects lung structure and gas exchange;
- at Key Stage 4 (14–16-year-olds) how solvents, tobacco, alcohol and other drugs affect bodily functions.

Curriculum guidance (DfE & School Curriculum and Assessment Authority, 1995) advises that in order to underpin effective approaches to drug education, schools need to have policies for drug education and for managing drug-related incidents. These will ensure a co-ordinated and consistent approach to drug education with clearly defined aims and objectives. The Office for Standards in Education (OFSTED) is charged with monitoring school policies and practice. Findings from visits in 1996 are available (OFSTED, 1997a, b).

Outside school

While a great deal of drug education and prevention work is done in schools, young people who are excluded or absent from school – over school-age – or in college, training or looking for work, are also targets for drug education and prevention. OFSTED conducted an evaluation of youth service provision for drug education with a particular focus on good practice. A report of their findings is available (OFSTED, 1997a).

There are no guidelines as such for drug education and prevention work that takes place outside the school setting.

The following approaches to drug education and prevention have been identified (Coggans & Watson, 1995):

- information based;
- values and skills based;
- resistance training;
- alternatives based;
- peer led.

In practice, these approaches are often combined, sometimes in a whole-school or whole-community approach to health education. But they are not always evaluated, and are not regulated or consistent either within localities or nationally.

Professional training

The training of professionals affects the type of drug education and prevention that is delivered. Many professionals who come into contact with young people will be expected to address drug use in the course of their work. The importance of providing relevant training has been underlined by the recent Department of Health Task Force review (Department of Health, 1996), which made the following recommendations:

- Professional bodies should review the extent to which they have implemented the ACMD's 1990 recommendations. These recommendations identified specific tasks for the medical, pharmaceutical, nursing, psychological, youth and community work, prison, police, and social work and probation sectors, as well as for the non-statutory sector, in implementing training on drugs and alcohol at undergraduate, postgraduate and post-qualification levels.

- Purchasers should require providers to examine levels of staff working with drug misusers and make sure that service budgets include enough to enable the right training to be undertaken (Department of Health, 1996, p. 92).

National and local support

The extent of national and local support for drug education and prevention affects the provision and type of initiatives that are developed. A number of agencies have a particular national or local remit for supporting the development of drug education and prevention. This remit is set out in *Tackling Drugs Together*.

For example, SCODA has a national remit with regard to drug services across the spectrum of drug education, prevention, treatment and care. Its role is to improve service provision by levering resources into the field; setting and promoting standards; monitoring and informing national and other policy; promoting good practice; and sharing ideas, skills, experiences, information and concerns.

Local support and expertise in drug education and prevention is provided in some areas by Home Office drug prevention teams. These teams work with their local communities in 12 areas in partnership with a wide range of other agencies and groups to develop effective ways of preventing the spread of drug misuse. The Home Office Drugs Prevention Initiative has published evaluation reports of local initiatives, and is committed to the dissemination of wide-ranging good practice guidelines based on its current programme of community based work. Where Home Office drug prevention teams do not exist, other local networks on prevention have often developed.

Drug Action Teams (DATs), advised by Drug Reference Groups (DRGs), are responsible locally for ensuring that government strategy on drug education and prevention is implemented. The focus of DATs is on improving community safety by reducing drug-related crime; and on reducing the susceptibility of young people to drug misuse, as well as reducing the health risks and other damage associated with drug misuse. These forums pool agency knowledge and expertise to assess local need, agree priorities and ensure that plans are put into action.

Funding

The purchasing and funding of drug education and prevention can be a key factor in the aims, content, methods, duration, quality and effectiveness of a programme. Education and prevention agencies may need to 'package' and redefine their services according to the philosophies and criteria of funders, and to meet local needs.

References

Coggans, N. & Watson, J. (1995) *Drug education: approaches, effectiveness and implications for delivery*. Health Education Board for Scotland, Edinburgh.

Department for Education (1995) *Drug prevention and schools*. Circular number 4/95.

Department for Education and the School Curriculum and Assessment Authority (1995) *Drug education: curriculum guidance for schools*.

Department of Health (1996) *The task force to review services for drug misusers: report of an independent review of drug treatment services in England*. HMSO.

Health Advisory Service (1996) *Children and young people: substance misuse services, the substance of young needs.* HMSO, London.

Home Office (1984) *Prevention: report of the Advisory Council on the Misuse of Drugs*. HMSO, London.

Office for Standards in Education (1997a) *The contribution of youth services to drug education*. HMSO, London.

Office for Standards in Education (1997b) *Drug education in schools*. HMSO, London.

Tackling Drugs Together – a strategy for England 1995–98 (1995). HMSO, London.

Chapter 2

Research methodology

Introduction

The HEA Drugs Team and SCODA undertook the Drug Education and Prevention Mapping Project between February and September 1996 to collect data on activities and organisations related to drug education and prevention. The decision was taken to use a three-part strategy, examining local activities, generic and specialist bodies, and national agencies, and to publish this information as a handbook for the purchasers and providers of prevention activity, DATs, DRGs and non-drug specialist professionals and agencies.

Research methods

The three-part strategy involved:

- Strand 1: a survey of 300 specific local drug education and prevention activities;
- Strand 2: a survey and analysis of the roles of generic and specialist local bodies in drug education and prevention work;
- Strand 3: an analysis of the roles of national and regional agencies in drug education and prevention.

This strategy is shown below as a pyramid, illustrating the three strands mapped by this work to represent the delivery and support of drug education and prevention.

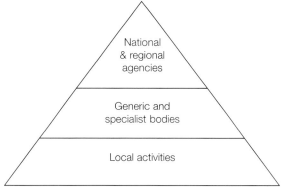

Figure 1 Pyramid structure of drug education and prevention activity at the level of local activities, generic and specialist bodies and national agencies

Criteria for inclusion

It was recognised at the outset that this first mapping project and handbook could only provide a 'snapshot of a field in motion'. As demonstrated by the mapping project, there are a great range of organisations involved in drug education and prevention, and there are many types of activities taking place. For this reason, criteria needed to be established for the mapping of Strand 1, in order to focus the scope of the project on just 300 local activities. These activities form the Directory section of this handbook (see page 65).

The survey was restricted to activities that included amongst their aims:

- reducing the incidence of drug use by preventing those people who have never used drugs, or who use them experimentally, from becoming or continuing as users;
- minimising harm related to the use of substances.

However, these aims are very broad and shared by a wide range of different organisations and activities. Further restrictions on activities for inclusion were made by specifying that they should be delivered directly to young people aged 11 to 25 or to those who will themselves directly deliver education and prevention messages to young people (see Figure 2).

Many activities therefore fell outside the scope of the project, such as:

- services for children and adults dealing principally in the care, treatment and rehabilitation of people who depend on, or misuse, substances;
- drug education that takes place as part of the school curriculum;
- physical resources used in drug education and prevention, such as training packs, leaflets and posters;
- community safety initiatives;
- enforcement measures that prevent the use of drugs, including market disruption, removal of drug users and dealers from circulation, physical design deterrents to drug using and dealing;
- professional training.

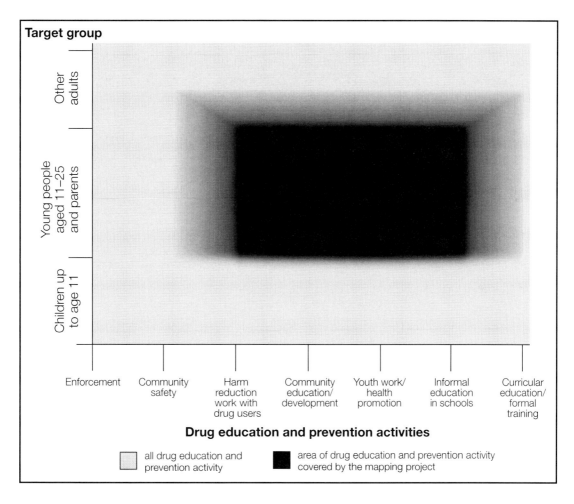

Figure 2 Drug education and prevention activity covered by the mapping project in relation to drug education and prevention as a whole

Data collection

The following describes the research undertaken in each of the three strands, and the additional information compiled.

Local activities

To undertake the mapping of local activities, 'snowballing' strategies were employed amongst drug services, DATs, police forces and drug prevention teams. This involved asking respondents for contact details of any organisations they knew to be undertaking drug education and prevention work. Criteria for inclusion in the mapping project were devised, and questionnaires sent to some 380 organisations in order to obtain details about the required 300 local activities.

Questionnaires returned (over 70%) were then checked against the criteria and for accuracy and omissions, and contact people were telephoned where necessary for further information. Information from the questionnaires was entered into a purpose-built database, which was cleaned and sorted to produce detailed indexes by organisation, activity, geographical location and DAT area.

In order to provide an insight into the practical implementation of local activities and their diversity, a number of projects were invited to expand upon the information supplied in their questionnaires. This was achieved through telephone and face-to-face interviews and the use of background literature.

Generic and specialist local bodies

Examples of rural, urban and rural/urban mix areas were researched. Over 40 local professionals and workers were interviewed by telephone and asked about their services, statutory responsibilities, expertise in drug education and prevention, and involvement in networks, forums and local planning. From this it was possible to build up a picture of what role each generic and specialist local body plays in drug education and prevention. The interviews were then transcribed, analysed and each body's role described.

National agencies

To identify the roles of national agencies in drug education and prevention, representatives from 16 national and regional agencies were visited and interviewed. One agency representative was telephone interviewed and written information was collated from four agencies. Respondents were asked the same questions as the generic and specialist local bodies. The interviews were then transcribed, information was extracted on each agency and each was sent a draft to check and edit.

Additional information

Several national funding sources were contacted, reviewed and their criteria summarised.

The Institute for the Study of Drug Dependence (ISDD) library undertook a literature search. Researchers collated information on other directories and literature mentioned by interviewees and mapping respondents during the research. Some of this information has been listed and is included in Appendix 2.

Chapter 3

Drug education and prevention in practice: examples of local activities

Introduction

The local activities included in this chapter have been taken from the Directory of local organisations and activities (see page 65). They have been expanded upon to provide a greater insight into the practical implementation of drug education and prevention work in the field. This 'snapshot' gives an impression of the diversity of projects running at any one time and which, for example, target specific population groups; have been set up after needs assessment; have a monitoring and evaluation component; support parents in working with young people; work in partnerships; are innovative or include an accreditation element.

Meeting the needs of the target group

Dance Drug Safety, Preston

Dance Drug Safety, run by Drugline Lancashire, based in Preston, is a project targeted at gay men. With very limited funds (£1250) it is run in both heterosexual and gay clubs and pubs in Preston and Blackpool. Features of the project include:

- maintaining a low-profile presence by staff members and volunteers in pubs and clubs, displaying posters, making leaflets available, and wearing T-shirts with an appropriate (to the target group) and subtle project logo;
- involving pub and club owners at the ideas stage of the project;
- involving gay men working in the field, and gay pub and club owners, in the setting up and carrying out of the project;
- encouraging involvement and awareness amongst pub and club staff and bouncers;
- setting realistic project aims, namely of harm prevention for people who regularly engage in dance drug and legal substance misuse;
- undertaking a needs assessment for the project, carried out by a forum of gay men;

- compiling an evaluation report of the work targeted at gay men, identifying the types of drugs gay men were using in clubs; their views on the project materials; the types of drug services they would use; the types of information needed for gay men;
- adopting a community development approach, which involves working in collaboration with other agencies.

For further information contact the Community Development Team: Tel. 01772 253840.

Frontline Peer Education Drug Project, Derby

The Frontline Peer Education Drug Project is a peer education project aimed at African Caribbean and Asian young people. It has one intake of 15 volunteers a year, for three years, from 1997–99. It is run by the Phoenix Project, Derby, which is a community health project set up to work with African Caribbean and Asian communities on issues of drugs, sexual health and alcohol.

The peer education programme is delivered from a black perspective, a major part of which involves discussing the negative stereotypes that exist about black people in relation to drug use and drug dealing. In order to promote a black perspective:

- all project workers are black;
- the curriculum is centred around black people's experiences of drug culture;
- peer educators are encouraged to deliver drug education in ways appropriate to their culture: for example, one of the volunteers uses rap music to communicate drug awareness messages.

For further information contact Leona Stanley: Tel. 01332 294898.

Young Women's Drug Project, Warmley

The Young Women's Drug Project is designed to raise young women's drugs awareness and to create drugs publicity and information written by young women for young women. It is run by the Clocktower Project (named after the building where the project is based) in Warmley, South Gloucestershire. The Clocktower Project is a young women's project in the Kingswood area, and is the only building in the area purpose-designed for young women.

Developing the Young Women's Drug Project involved visiting local youth clubs (usually on a 'girls' night'), showing young women the information already produced by the project, and involving them in discussions on a planned booklet and on whether they agreed or disagreed with the aims of the project. Some 13 young women decided to attend the sessions, and they participated in the development of the Sorting Out Drugs Awareness (SODA) booklet from October 1994 to March 1995. This involved attending a two-hour session one night a week for six months.

A typical session comprised:

- a half-hour chat;
- a one-hour planning/organising/discussion session;
- a half-hour wind-down.

The first session included:

- addressing ideas such as 'drugs are a male issue', looking at participants' own drug use and how young women feel about drugs;
- talking about the purpose of the project and where the funding originated, and agreeing aims;
- deciding what the participants thought they needed and wanted from a publication.

Positive effects on the young women involved in the project meant that some went on to speak to their school class about the project, how it was run and the publication they developed. Other participants used their experience to inform their college portfolio.

One measure of the effectiveness of the project in empowering participants to express themselves about drugs is that the outcome was different from the project workers' plan. A leaflet had been proposed, but a 24-page booklet was the outcome.

The project worker and participants disseminated the booklet to schools, voluntary youth groups, youth clubs and health visitors, using interest gained in the booklet to attract a new group of women to the drug project.

Other drug education and prevention projects being planned by the Clocktower Project include a young women's drugs drop-in service, called Sisters in the Hood.

For further information contact Tina Bond: Tel. 0117 967 1655.

Delivering drug education to a rural community

West Sussex Rural Youth Mobile Project, Petworth

West Sussex Rural Youth Mobile Project provides a youth service, information, and a social venue in villages with little or no active youth provision. The professional management of the project is the responsibility of the rural development worker supported by the steering group, which comprises West Sussex Youth Service, Sussex Rural Community Council, representatives of local communities and young people.

The need for the mobile was established by youth workers and volunteers asking young people what kind of facility was needed, what they thought of the idea of a bus, and how they thought it could be used. The bus facilities and activities are aimed at young people aged 13 to 18; it operates five nights a week for two hours from 8 pm to 10 pm (different villages each night), and is staffed by two youth workers.

The aim of the work centred on the bus is to minimise the harm that legal and illegal substances can do, and to get young people involved in activities which divert them from using substances.

Drug education is provided in the context of general health education and of decision making and life skills education, as it was not seen as being desirable or useful for rural communities to regard the bus as a 'drugs bus'.

The work that goes on in or around the bus is often activity centred: role-plays, games, quizzes and questionnaires are used, and barbecues and outdoor sports are also organised.

It takes a long time to build up relationships with young people, even if a local worker is invited on board to 'bridge the gap' and speed up the process, so the bus needs to visit a particular village every week for a minimum of 12 weeks.

The bus does not visit any one village for more than 20 weeks, as another aim is to encourage young people to set up their own activities and projects, or a meeting place for themselves after the bus has stopped visiting. It does revisit from time to time to check on progress and to provide support.

For further information contact Maureen Sargent: Tel. 01798 342547.

Developing guidance

SHED, Sheffield

SHED offer a Safer Dancing Service to clubs that advertise dance nights with music such as Jungle, Happy Hardcore, Techno, Garage, Trance, Ambient and House.

Before they established this service, they carried out research amongst clubbers in four major venues in Sheffield to find out their average age, how often they went out, if they used dance drugs and if they would like access to drug workers at an event or venue. As a result of this research, SHED was able to draw up a number of recommendations to club owners for safer dancing.

The research, carried out between February and April 1996, based upon data collected from 674 clubbers (which represents approximately 15% of clubbers in Sheffield), demonstrated that:

- the majority of clubbers (78%) have at some point used drugs in clubs;
- 38% of those questioned attend clubs weekly and 29% use drugs in clubs on a weekly basis;
- 80% of those questioned would like drug workers available at clubs and events;
- the media focus on ecstasy did not seem to have impacted greatly on people's drug use: clubbers argued that media reports were sensationalist and misinformed, and expressed concern about the lack of reliable, up-to-date, unbiased information on drugs available to young people. A minority had reduced or ceased their use of ecstasy, but in many cases this had been replaced by the use of other substances such as amphetamines and alcohol.

Based on the survey information, client work and professional judgement, project workers recommended that clubs should:

- employ Safer Dancing Initiatives via their local drug agencies;
- provide up-to-date harm-reduction drugs literature to customers;
- provide free water, adequate ventilation and sufficient chill-out areas with seating;
- train security staff to recognise drugs problems and to treat people appropriately.

These recommendations are echoed in recent Home Office guidance on conditions for licences to pubs and clubs.

For further information contact Anna Christophorou/Janine Scorthorne: Tel. 0114 272 9164.

Obtaining feedback and implementing monitoring and evaluation

Parents for Prevention, Birmingham

Initially, Parents for Prevention provided comment sheets for parents, asking them to give feedback on the sessions in which they participated. However, they found that parents did not always write down what they thought. Now they always incorporate a 'closing round' during the talk, when staff ask parents to make three comments each. Written evaluation sheets are still used when the group is large.

More details about Parents for Prevention are given in the section on Drug Awareness Talks on page 19.

Drugline Lancashire, Preston

Drugline Lancashire monitors and evaluates its drugs awareness education events in the following ways.

Efforts are made to record every educational session that is held throughout the year, the numbers of participants at each event, and whether they are adults or young people. The figures are collated monthly or annually.

Attempts to evaluate the quality and usefulness of events are always made: a feedback questionnaire is handed out for participants to fill in and verbal feedback is encouraged. Past findings include fear and concern over drug use, and misunderstandings of both the suitability of agencies and how to gain access to them.

The feedback received is used to inform the fundraising priorities for developing the project; objectives include the need to continually develop and update teaching methods and materials in order that drugs awareness sessions continue to be attractive to young people; and the need to enhance service accessibility to young people.

More details about Drugline Lancashire are given in the section on Dance Drug Safety on page 13.

Reaching young people through their parents

Drug Awareness Talks, Birmingham

Drug Awareness Talks for parents are run by Parents for Prevention in Birmingham. This organisation was set up in 1994 to:

- educate parents, including helping them to feel more confident and reassured about drugs and their effects and about providing support to young people;
- provide support to parents who are having to deal with their own or their children's drug-related problems.

Drug Awareness Talks are organised in response to organisations or groups seeking Parents for Prevention's help with drug education and prevention. Requests come from residents' associations, neighbourhood offices, community groups, schools, governors and parent–teacher associations. In response, staff (and often parent volunteers) arrange to hold a talk after establishing what kind of drug education the group is requesting.

At the beginning of a talk the aims, objectives and agenda are established with the group attending. The presentation depends on the number of parents attending: if there are over 30, staff and volunteers are limited as to how far participants can be involved; a group of between six and eight is often the most productive and rewarding for participants.

Themes covered in the talks include:

- drugs, their effects, and what they look like;
- the nature and effect of people's drug use;
- advice to parents on what to do if they have a child showing signs of problems with drugs;
- what Parents for Prevention can do to support them in that event;
- how to educate children by building self-confidence and encouraging decision-making skills;
- the advantages and disadvantages of encouraging children to take risks;
- the management of substances in the home (from medicines to alcohol and tobacco);
- at what age drug education can start.

Parents for Prevention volunteers often attend talks; this provides the participants with the opportunity to talk to them individually about specific problems they may face. The organisation also runs 'Living with Teenagers' support groups. These can be useful as a mechanism for parents to begin discussing their own substance use.

For further information contact Rosie Higgins: Tel. 0121 454 5805.

Parents Against Drug Abuse

Parents Against Drug Abuse (PADA) run a national annual parents convention to which they invite existing parents' groups, groups that are starting up, and parents from areas where such groups do not exist. The convention takes place over a one- or two-day period. Professionals and outside speakers are deliberately not invited. However, a minister is invited to attend and listen to parents' views. In 1996 Tom Sackville, MP, attended.

PADA also acts as an umbrella organisation for other parents' groups, offering advice on how to start up, set up a constitution and gain funding.

For further information contact Joan Keogh: Tel. 0151 652 9108.

Funding projects through the Single Regeneration Budget

SHED, Sheffield

Single Regeneration Budget (SRB) funding which is provided by regional government offices, has been accessed by SHED in Sheffield to develop drug education for young people sessions with the local groups that request them. Volunteers run a number of sessions with youth groups, children's units and schools, making themselves available to answer questions about drugs. If desired by the group, SHED develops further drug education and prevention work with them. Past activities include a drama workshop and peer education training.

SHED's bid for SRB funds was assisted by the fact that Sheffield's theme at the time of the bid was 'Young People and the Community'. Applicants for SRB funding must match the budget they are given, and SHED was successful in gaining this financial help from the police authority, the regional health authority, Safer Cities and Joint Finance.

Another requirement of SRB funding is that data collection and monitoring take place while the project is being carried out. This involves the production of monthly reports showing, for instance, milestones achieved, the number of people contacted and the number of sessions held by project workers. Annual appraisals are also held with the project workers, and annual funding may not be made available until the appraisal is satisfactorily completed. See page 306 for further information on SRB funding.

SHED is a young people's drug project based at the Rockingham Drug Project, Sheffield. Its services include education, counselling and support, work with young people who are in trouble with the law, a Safer Dancing Service (see Developing Guidance on page 17) and outreach.

For further information contact Susie Sykes: Tel. 0114 272 9164.

The role of information technology

Information and Advice, Norwich

Information and Advice is provided by the Mancroft Advice Project to young people aged 16 to 26 in Norwich. The project has a purpose-built drop-in centre offering advice and information to young people. The largest area of its work is counselling.

The project is currently developing its provision of drug education and local service information via an interactive computer package aimed at young people leaving home. The package is designed to give information on all aspects of leaving home, and has its origins in the Centrepoint Leaving Home Partnership Group. It will be available to youth centres and clubs, Citizens Advice Bureaux, schools, social services and other agencies for the cost of a computer disc.

The package can be used on IBM-compatible PCs and Apple Macintosh computers, and is designed to be used by young people with little or no knowledge of computers. By touching a map and typing a topic, users can access a screen of information about the topic and a list of services in the area.

One of the major benefits of the project is its potential to deliver information and advice to the rural areas of Norfolk; for example by being available in local youth clubs. In October 1996 a pilot version was tested with young people, and the package adapted according to feedback. The launch of the full package was scheduled for April 1997.

For further information contact Peter Bainbridge: Tel. 01603 766994.

Setting up a drug-free venue

Youth Trust, Barnstaple

The Youth Trust in Barnstaple is developing the Inn, which aims to provide an alternative place for young people aged 13 to 25 to go.

The Inn will provide the following drug education and prevention services:

- a drug-free meeting place for young people aged 13 to 17 who are too young to go into pubs or clubs, and so presently congregate on the streets, where they are vulnerable;
- training in a range of skills and activities for young people up to the age of 25 to help build a sense of self-esteem, including skills learned in managing the Inn;
- training for a selected group of young people in peer education techniques, enabling them to educate their friends and colleagues in the dangers of drug use.

The project is founded on the belief that:

- attempts to solve the drug problem by controlling supply are doomed to failure: the only way forward is by working to reduce the demand for illegal drugs;
- attempts by adults to dissuade young people from experimenting with drugs ('Just say no') are futile and counterproductive;
- any solution needs to be guided by young people for young people.

The Youth Trust has a Young Management Team who are closely involved in designing the Inn. The first facility to be provided will be a coffee bar, with further phases of development including:

- workshops in music, art, theatre and photography;
- a recording studio;
- a live music venue;
- a restaurant.

One of the main factors leading to the creation of the project was consultation with the police and local drugs rehabilitation centre, which identified £22.5 million of drug-related crime annually in north Devon. Benefits to the whole community are anticipated from a reduction in drug-related crime, and the fear of such crime.

For further information contact Will Palin: Tel. 01271 321100.

Giving awards for drug prevention

Duke of Westminster's Award for Services in Drug Prevention, Birkenhead

The Duke of Westminster's Award for Services in Drug Prevention is run annually by Parents Against Drug Abuse (PADA), based in the Wirral.

An annual competition has been held since 1993, in which groups or individuals who have made an outstanding achievement in drug prevention are invited to take part. Leaflets about the scheme are distributed to local schools and youth clubs during the summer to make them aware of the competition.

All those applying for the award need to be nominated by a friend, teacher, parent, youth worker or anyone who knows about the applicant(s) and the project undertaken. Nomination forms are sent to all those who express an interest in the award.

Winners of the award in previous years have been:

- three young women aged 17 to 18 who gave lessons about drugs in school;
- Kids Against Drugs, who carried out a Drug Free School project;
- Bromley Youth Centre, which made a video containing anti-drugs messages;
- a young woman who designed an anti-drugs poster featuring a pair of scales and the caption 'You are worth more than drugs'.

The number of applications for the award increases each year the scheme is run, with more than 200 received for the 1995–6 round.

The organisers of the winning projects receive a cash prize of up to £250; a framed certificate signed by the founder of PADA, Joan Keogh; and a plaque and silver cup engraved with their name which they can keep for 12 months, until the next award.

The award ceremony takes place at a charity evening held at Eaton Hall near Chester, where the winners are presented with their awards by the Duke of Westminster.

The effects of the award scheme (identified by PADA) on the individuals or groups participating include:

- making them more interested in the dangers of drug use;
- spreading anti-drugs messages amongst their friends;
- gaining experience of organising and running a small project; making them aware of PADA, its rationale and how it works.

One member of an award winning group went on to complete two weeks of vocational training with PADA, and demonstrated an interest in pursuing a career working in the drugs prevention field.

Further information about PADA is given under Parents Against Drug Abuse on page 20.

Accreditation of peer educators

African Caribbean and Asian Peer Education, Leicester

African Caribbean and Asian Peer Education is one of the projects run by the Leicester Drug Advice Centre. The centre provides free confidential help and advice on drugs and drug problems.

Accreditation of volunteer peer educators' learning is provided by the Open College Network. To gain accreditation status for the programme the organisers contacted the Open College Network and described the course they wanted to run. They were allocated a worker from the college, who helped them set out the programme organisation and delivery. This needed to be sub-divided into 'units', which are discrete episodes of learning designed to be taken in order and to build upon each other. The accreditation requires each unit to have a title, pre-determined outcomes, criteria for assessment, a credit level and number of credits section. A submission document is then drawn up and approved by the college.

Units that potential peer educators can take on the African Caribbean and Asian Peer Education programme are:

- personal development;
- street drugs awareness;

- society, drugs and black communities;
- peer education facilitator skills.

Each unit has a credit level which is equivalent to NVQ levels 1, 2 or 3 and can be used to access further education.

For further information contact Deborah Sangster: Tel. 0116 247 0200.

Chapter 4

The role of generic and specialist local bodies

Introduction

The following summaries are derived from the research into the role of generic and specialist local drug education and prevention services. Three geographic areas were examined as examples of rural, rural/urban and urban environments. The results illustrate a slice of the drug education and prevention strategy and networking that occurs throughout England. Due to the recent establishment of Drug Action Teams (DATs) and Drug Reference Groups (DRGs), and to the redrawing of local and health authority boundaries and roles, many drug education and prevention networks in these areas are in the process of readjustment.

Community safety and development bodies

Community safety forums and partnerships provide the opportunity for a wide variety of local services and corporate representatives to share ideas and views, and to form plans of action with regard to community safety and development in their locality. Membership may include representatives from community development, crime prevention, housing, planning, environment, police, social services, probation, the health authority, the Local Education Authority (LEA) and local business. Although these bodies have no specific responsibilities for drug education and prevention, they regard both as important means of reducing drug-related crime. These forums and partnerships often initiate and facilitate inter-agency projects, as in the case of one community safety forum that initiated a young persons' information and advice project which included drug information. In some areas local authorities set up specific community safety units to deal with drug education and prevention.

Some community safety forums are based in community development or environment departments which, though they have no statutory responsibilities regarding drug education and prevention, may support this through their outreach work, or through multi-agency health promotion partnerships. One such department provides field-worker support for a parent-run drug education and prevention organisation; another trains its outreach workers in drug education and prevention techniques through its in-house training programme.

Drug Action Teams (DATs) and Drug Reference Groups (DRGs)

Each DAT and DRG reflects the circumstances of its specific geographical area, but is driven by the same underlying purpose in terms of drug education and prevention, community safety and treatment issues: namely, to co-ordinate greater inter-agency dialogue, thereby identifying local needs and developing a strategic plan which addresses these needs and avoids duplication of services. This purpose is illustrated by the action of one DRG which recognised an inconsistency in drug education and prevention work in local schools due to the number of independent and grant-maintained schools in the region. It proposed the establishment of a local forum of teachers from every school through which a consistent plan could be developed for drug education and prevention in all schools, not only those under the jurisdiction of the LEA.

DAT and DRG members represent a broad range of services, thus forming a considerable body of expertise in both drug education and prevention and in related areas. The configuration of specialist and non-specialist agencies within DATs and DRGs varies widely around the country.

Since DATs exist as co-ordinating bodies, they do not provide direct client services. Some appoint co-ordinators, while others use the funding for servicing meetings and research projects. However, they can access funding for DAT-initiated and inter-agency projects primarily from the budgets of represented individual local agencies, and also from the Challenge Fund (Central Drugs Co-ordination Unit). Other indirect sources of funding are: the Department for Education and Employment (DfEE) Grants for Education Support and Training (GEST) funding, the Single Regeneration Budget (SRB), and European funding.

Middlesex University Social Policy Research Centre has conducted an interim assessment of the development of 105 DATs in England. Findings are reported in Tackling Drugs Locally (HMSO, 1997).

Drug services: non-statutory and voluntary

Non-statutory drug services offer a wide range of services in drug education and prevention, including schools work, outreach, drop-in information centres and counselling. They are frequently more involved in drug education and prevention than statutory drug agencies, which are usually treatment oriented. Staff are often well trained in youth work, drug issues and educative work. They often provide training for the staff of non-specialist agencies, and are involved in inter-agency programmes in schools.

Non-statutory drug services are funded mainly by health authorities, and to a lesser extent by local authorities, and also receive funding from charitable foundations. They can apply for further funding for special projects from the health authority and trust funds, and through partnership bids. Some services have identified a need for outreach work for stimulant users, since centre-based work tends to focus on opiate use. They have obtained funding for projects which take place in mobile units, pubs and clubs, often using peer educators and volunteers.

Non-statutory drug services are closely linked with other agencies, both through referrals and collaborative projects. They work closely with schools, education advisers, police and Health Promotion Units (HPUs). Some non-statutory drug services network with other non-statutory bodies through a committee of welfare organisations. Most non-statutory drug services access the DAT or DRG through their local health authority contact. Although drug services in the voluntary sector currently have the second largest representation on DRGs, overall there is little direct input into DAT or DRG networks at present.

GPs

As GPs work on an individual client basis, their involvement in drug education and prevention varies, and is dependent on the needs of the particular client and the discretion of the GP. GPs refer clients to local drug services for further treatment or information, when appropriate, or upon the request of the client. Some GPs further their knowledge of drug issues through professional development courses in health promotion or through drug-specific courses.

Extra funding may be available for practices to run projects which target specific issues. One example of this involves a practice which works with homeless people, in conjunction with the Salvation Army, and specifically addresses drug and alcohol issues. Individual GPs may liaise with local drug workers and drug agencies, and often sit on steering committees of voluntary organisations or local agencies. They may be represented on the DAT and DRG through a member of the local medical committee or GP forum, and in this way can contribute and advise on local drug education and prevention planning.

Health authorities

The role of the health authority is largely one of commissioning and purchasing services. Consequently, its strategies serve to direct local planning. Although a significant proportion of health authority funding targets treatment services, there is an emphasis both on primary prevention and harm minimisation in terms of drug use. Health authorities seek to develop an effective and consistent purchasing strategy which is relevant to their community. They may do this by:

- establishing the precise needs of their community through DATs, DRGs and commissioned research;
- making funding choices which avoid duplication or omission of services;
- monitoring and evaluating existing health authority funded agencies;
- fostering a multi-agency approach by writing the appropriate caveats into their funding agreements.

Not only do health authorities link into local networks through representation on the DATs and DRGs, but, by virtue of their role as chief funding body, they also have direct contact with all statutory and most non-statutory agencies. They work closely with education advisers and youth and community services, usually approaching drug education and prevention from a health promotion perspective. One health authority has established a post specifically to liaise with the voluntary sector. By so doing, the health authority hopes to strengthen links with voluntary sector drug education and prevention providers, build trust and inform its purchasing decisions. In many regions the prevailing strategies of the health authority are a determining factor in local drug education and prevention planning.

Health education advisers

LEA health education advisers are responsible for co-ordinating drug education and prevention work in schools. This involves policy making, developing a cohesive programme between all primary and secondary schools, and liaising with teachers, police, the health authority and Health Promotion Unit. It may also include working with parents and co-ordinating drug education and prevention in youth and community groups. For instance, one health education adviser took the opportunity to reinforce the schools drug education and prevention programme through outreach work undertaken by voluntary agencies, and thus to provide a homogeneous approach to drug education and prevention to young people of all ages.

Health education advisers come from a variety of specialist backgrounds. They are often teachers with expertise in health education and subsequent training in drug awareness, and are frequently called upon to run courses on drug education and prevention for parents, teachers and voluntary organisations. The health education adviser posts are funded by the LEA, and further funding for specific projects is available through GEST funds, the LEA and local sources.

Health education advisers work closely with Health Promotion Units, especially in areas where there is a Healthy Schools initiative. They maintain close links with services which provide drug education and prevention in schools. In some areas, these groups have formed a charter by which all agencies who take part in school-based drug education and prevention work must agree to certain policies and procedures, with the aim of standardising the quality of drug education and prevention in schools across the region. Health education advisers are often central to local inter-agency dialogue. They are involved with the National Health Education Liaison Group, and sit on local drugs forums and DRGs, accessing the DATs through their LEA representative.

Health Promotion Units

Health Promotion Units (HPUs) encourage people to make informed choices with regard to their drug-related behaviour. These units are funded by health authorities and may act as resource and referral agencies, foster schools work and peer education programmes, or core-fund voluntary agencies on behalf of the health authority. Staff in the units generally have training in specific health issues, experience in the health service and expertise in needs assessment.

HPU-funded programmes centre on providing health information, building life skills and enhancing personal and social development. HPU officers work closely with local schools, Local Education Authority (LEA) advisers and teachers. In some instances these collaborations result in the implementation of the Healthy Schools award and other such programmes.

The role of the HPU in local drug education and prevention work varies between health authorities. In one example, the HPU serves only as a resource centre for drug education and prevention information, since the work of two local drug services obviated the need for a greater role. In another example, the HPU is involved in establishing a multi-agency health promotion project which serves as a forum for local health planning. In addition to involvement with other health networks, HPUs are linked to DATs and DRGs through health authority representatives.

Home Office Drugs Prevention Initiative (DPI) teams

From 1990 to 1995 there were small Home Office DPI teams in 20 separate areas. Since April 1995, 12 larger teams have covered a wider area in England. Until 1999 the work of individual teams will be funded, supported and co-ordinated by the Central Drugs Prevention Unit, based in the Home Office in London. See the entry in chapter 5 for more information about the work of the Home Office DPI.

NHS statutory drug agencies

NHS statutory drug agencies are heavily involved in drug treatment. However, they also contribute to drug education and prevention in varying capacities, which is dependent on funding, availability of other services and the prevailing policies of the NHS trust.

In most cases, NHS statutory drug agencies have very little funding available for primary drug prevention, focusing on treatment-based education and secondary prevention amongst existing service users. Nevertheless these agencies use their medical and treatment expertise to contribute to the drug education and prevention networks in other ways: for example, by belonging to local planning and strategy committees, giving advice on drug education and prevention documents and materials, and developing local strategy and running courses for non-drug specialists. One treatment-based statutory drug agency provides a nurse who specialises in harm minimisation with pregnant women.

Other NHS statutory drug agencies have a more specific brief with regard to drug education and prevention, often reflecting a deficit of drug education and prevention work provided by local agencies. These statutory drug agencies may support work in schools, co-ordinate inter-agency work in the area and work with social services and youth services. Some actively participate, in collaboration with the health education adviser, in drug education and prevention work and programme development in schools. NHS statutory drug agencies have links with local agencies through the DRG and are represented on various other drugs forums, with respect both to treatment and education.

Police services

The police service has a high profile in the provision of drug education and prevention, particularly in schools. Some forces adopt a philosophy of harm minimisation without compromising their stance against drug-related crime. Drug education officers take a wide variety of approaches in their work with parents, teachers, other police officers, students and community groups. In the case of schools work, one police service may train its officers in teaching skills, thus enabling them to run specific programmes in a classroom situation; another service may use officers who have a high level of knowledge in the drugs field to work with teachers, acting as a resource for teacher-led sessions. Both these approaches are, however, founded on the basic premise that the police service's expertise in drug education and prevention does not lie in the areas of counselling and teaching, but rather in a knowledge of the law, substances and contemporary drug culture.

Police services differ in their approaches, facilities and funding available for drug education and prevention. One service accesses money from a 'drug seizure' fund and from court awards. These funds are then used to sponsor research, training and prevention programmes, one of which was a Drugs In Sport conference.

Officers from the police services fulfil active roles in inter-agency work, and in particular with the LEA, youth and community services, and local drug agencies. One police service in the study operates an arrest referral scheme. Upon release, every arrestee is issued with information concerning drug use, and referral details for local drug agencies. Another service is party to the establishment of a 'schools charter' which standardises the practices of all those involved in drug education and prevention in schools. Such inter-agency links are enhanced by police representation on DATs.

Probation services

Although the remit of the probation service does not include a responsibility to provide drug education and prevention, there are instances of such education in individual cases. This may occur at the client's request, or in cases where drug use interferes with the client's probation status. While some probation officers may have training in drug treatment, most have no training in drug education and prevention, and will refer their clients to local drug services for further information and advice.

Probation services are usually closely linked with social services and local drug services. They use these drug services as a resource for their clients. Drug service staff frequently provide in-house training for probation officers. Links with drug education and prevention networks are provided by representation on DATs and DRGs. One probation service was involved in setting up a multi-agency working group to reduce drug-related crime, which led to the instigation of awareness training for magistrates, thereby ensuring more effective sentencing for drug-related crimes.

Social services

Social services operate in a wide variety of situations which involve adult care, accommodation for children in need, youth justice, and the parental responsibility for young people. Most of these situations incorporate individual client work, and include building life and social skills, as well as providing information which allows the client to make informed choices about their life. It is in this context that a social worker may provide information about drug education and prevention or refer the client to a specialist agency. In particular situations, social workers may prefer to use local drug services as a resource by which they access drug education and prevention information for themselves, and then impart it to their clients. This system is used to keep drug education and prevention within the bounds of a carefully established and delicately balanced trust relationship between the client and social worker.

Social services staff have specific skills in social work and communication. Some social services secure specific grants for alcohol and drugs work, but this is usually for treatment provision. Drug education and prevention work carried out by staff depends largely on client need, staff knowledge and confidence. Some staff have a special interest in drug education and prevention and receive in-house training in drug awareness and health education.

Social services may collaborate with local drugs agencies on joint partnership bids. They are represented on DATs and various other local planning committees.

Voluntary youth and education organisations

Voluntary youth and education organisations provide an important link with young people and community members whereby information regarding health, drugs and life skills can be accessed. This often takes place in the context of a drop-in centre, a theatre-in-education production, a mobile unit, or on the street, via an outreach worker. Drug education and prevention work may be undertaken by youth workers or peer educators. In many instances staff will refer young people to local drug services for more detailed drug education and prevention work.

Voluntary youth and education organisations are usually funded by local authority grants, charitable sources and occasionally private trusts, lottery grants, charity projects, or European funding. Their services are often purchased by youth services or LEAs. Representation on local planning committees and DRGs varies between organisations, but unless they are connected to a larger agency, it is often difficult for smaller voluntary organisations to have an input into local discussion. In one area, the local welfare organisations formed a committee which provided them with an opportunity to participate in local strategy, and led to a representative being invited on to the local DRG.

Youth services

Youth services vary widely in their approach to the provision of services. Some operate their youth projects by grant funding of non-statutory bodies. Most, however, balance the purchasing of specialist services with the direct provision of generic and specialist services. Although drugs work is not a statutory requirement of the youth service, many consider that drug education and prevention is an implicit responsibility in the social education and personal development of young people.

Some youth services train their youth staff in drug education and prevention and provide them with suitable materials to use in youth and outreach work. One youth service uses staff on secondment from HPUs for specific drug education and prevention work in youth centres. Youth workers refer young people to local specialist agencies, and often use resources from these agencies in youth clubs. In the case of youth services which function primarily through the grant funding of non-statutory bodies, youth worker training and practice is varied.

Youth services provide funding for non-statutory youth organisations, and seek funding for their own projects from local sources and partnership bids. They work with local drug services, HPUs, health authorities, social services and police in local planning organisations, and on joint drug education and prevention projects. One youth service informs its strategic planning through a forum of 100 young people drawn from youth clubs. The forum is used as a focus group by which the youth service establishes the perspectives and needs of young people in the area. Youth services also have links with other agencies through representation on DRGs and DATs.

Chapter 5

The role of national and regional agencies

Introduction

This chapter profiles 19 national agencies and one regional agency.

The information provided relates to each agency's role in drug education and prevention specifically, rather than their role in, for example, treatment and care, or criminal justice.

The range covered by the agencies is England only unless specified and five key identifiers have been used to categorise the agencies:

- forum   **F**
- government department   **GD**
- national voluntary organisation   **NVO**
- non-governmental organisation   **NGO**
- special health authority.   **SHA**

Association of Chief Police Officers (ACPO) Drugs Sub-Committee

Greater Manchester Police HQ
PO Box 22 (SW PDO)
Chester House, Boyer Street
Manchester M16 0RE
Tel: 0161 856 2029/2016
Fax: 0161 856 2036

For further information contact: Assistant Chief Constable Alan Castree, Honorary Secretary
Range: England and Wales

Services provided

Each of the 43 police forces in England and Wales is independent and has its own strategy on drugs within the framework provided by the White Paper *Tackling Drugs Together*. ACPO is an organisation that represents chief police officers for England and Wales; its role in the police force is to produce guidance on issues for police personnel. Its Drugs Sub-Committee focuses on drugs and has produced a drugs strategy for use by forces.

Expertise and special knowledge

ACPO draws on and shares the expertise of all its member forces. If educational material or research is produced by one force, this may be made available to other forces. Notifications of such work may be found in Home Office publications, which all forces receive.

Links with other agencies

ACPO has links with Customs and Excise, the prison service, the Department of Health, the Health Education Authority, the Doping Control Unit, SCODA, the Home Office Drugs Prevention Initiative, the Central Drugs Co-ordination Unit, and other local and voluntary agencies.

Involvement with other networks

ACPO is represented on the National Children's Bureau Drug Education Forum, the Local Government Drugs Forum and the Advisory Council on the Misuse of Drugs.

Central Drugs Co-ordination Unit (CDCU)

Room 67D/4
Government Offices
Great George Street
London SW1P 3AL
Tel: 0171 270 5776
Fax: 0171 270 5857

For further information contact: Liz Gass, Office Manager

Services provided

The CDCU is responsible for overseeing the implementation of the government's drugs strategy *Tackling Drugs Together* and for ensuring that all tasks in the strategy are carried out. It co-ordinates the work of government departments, facilitates and supports DATs, and puts enquirers in touch with other organisations or departments. The CDCU holds conferences for DAT co-ordinators and chairs, which enable them to share their experiences and network.

It has also commissioned two publications for DATs: a digest of good practice, which covers all areas of government policy, including education; and *Tackling Drugs Informatively*, which advises DATs of local and national information sources on drugs. The CDCU also commissioned *Tackling Drugs Locally*, which is an interim assessment of the development of 105 DATs in England.

Funding available

The CDCU co-ordinated the Challenge Funding bids from DATs.

Links with other agencies

The CDCU works with all departments, organisations and individuals involved in the *Tackling Drugs Together* strategy. In education and prevention in particular it has close links with the Department of Health (DoH) and the Department for Education and Employment (DfEE).

Involvement with other networks

The CDCU has observer status on the National Children's Bureau Drug Education Forum.

Involvement in local planning

Much of the work of the CDCU is in supporting DATs to implement the drugs strategy at local level. DAT action plans were submitted to the CDCU at the end of 1995. The Lord President approved all plans by April 1996. DAT revised action plans for 1997/8 were submitted at the end of April 1997, and were approved by the President, the Right Honourable Ann Taylor MP. Visits are made from the CDCU to all DATs, at least annually, to gather information about good practice and to offer information and advice to DATs.

Department for Education and Employment (DfEE)

Health Education Team
Sanctuary Buildings
Great Smith Street
London SW1P 3BT
Tel: 0171 925 6302
Fax: 0171 925 6988

For further information contact: John Ford, Head of Personal, Social and Health Education Team

Services provided

The DfEE provides guidance, funding and support to local education authorities for local drug education and health education. Guidance was issued on drug prevention and schools in May 1995 (circular 4/95). Funding is provided through the GEST programme which supports two types of activity: teacher training on drugs, and innovative approaches to delivering drug education projects.

In 1995–6, 16 projects involving various innovative approaches to delivering drug education were funded. In 1996–7 eight of the above projects are continuing to be funded and ten new projects have been funded. In 1997–8 there will continue to be GEST funding available for both teacher training and other projects.

Projects funded through the grants programme are evaluated as part of OFSTED's schools inspection. In July 1996, the department held a national conference to disseminate the findings of the first year of projects (1995–6) and to present findings from OFSTED's evaluations.

The aim of the projects is to draw together information on methods of good practice on the delivery of drug education, and information will be disseminated in late 1997, when the department plans to issue a booklet detailing good practices from the projects.

Statutory responsibilities

There is a statutory requirement as part of the National Curriculum Science Order for schools to deliver drug education at each of the Key Stages 1–4 (spanning education for 5- to 16-year-olds).

This requirement represents the statutory minimum for schools. The department's responsibility is to see that the GEST programmes are undertaken and evaluated.

Expertise and special knowledge

The administrators within the department consult with experts, advisers and networks of specialists in the drug field and in education, including OFSTED, when drawing up its policies.

Funding available

GEST funding is available through competitive bids and includes a local education authority contribution. Some £6 million per year was spent on drug education and prevention in 1995/6 and 1996/7, which comprises £4.5 million for teacher training and £1.5 million for innovative projects. A similar total is expected to be available for 1997/8.

Links with other agencies

The DfEE sits on the Advisory Council on the Misuse of Drugs, on prevention working groups, and the statistics research committee. It liaises with all other government departments concerned in the *Tackling Drugs Together* strategy.

Involvement with other networks

The DfEE is represented on the Interdepartmental Group on Drugs and Solvents Publicity and is a member of the Council of Europe's Pompidou Group Prevention Working Party.

Involvement in local planning

If advice is sought, the department responds to queries or refers enquirers to other agencies.

Department of Health (DoH)

Wellington House
133–155 Waterloo Road
London SE1 8UG
Tel: 0171 972 4172
Fax: 0171 972 4198

For further information contact: Alastair Thomas, Drugs Prevention and Publicity Team, Health Promotion Division.

Services provided

The DoH commissions services and projects in England from national provider agencies. Those with drug education and prevention elements include:

- the Health Education Authority's contract to provide health promotion literature and publicity campaigns on drugs and solvent misuse;
- the National Drugs Helpline;
- Section 64 funding of: ADFAM National, apa (Association for the Prevention of Addiction), the Institute for the Study of Drug Dependence, the Solvent Abuse Resource Group (SARG), the Standing Conference on Drug Abuse (SCODA), TACADE, and Turning Point.

Statutory responsibilities

The DoH's role in drug education and prevention originates from a wider brief as set out in the 1919 Public Health Act, which is to protect public health. It also fulfils a major role in drug education and prevention as set out in the White Paper *Tackling Drugs Together*, namely to help young people to resist drugs and to reduce the health risks of drug misuse.

Expertise and special knowledge

The health promotion division of the DoH has specialist medical knowledge, experience of policy development, and knowledge of developing, implementing and evaluating drug education and prevention initiatives.

Funding available

Funding currently allocated for health promotion with regard to drugs is:

- £5 million a year on information provision and publicity campaigns;
- £1.3 million a year on the provision of both the National Drugs Helpline and the National AIDS Helpline;
- £1.7 million a year on Section 64 grants for projects.

These figures include funding for projects and organisations that work on the treatment aspect as well as the education and prevention aspect of drug misuse.

Links with other agencies

The department has working links with the Scottish and Welsh Offices and the Department of Health and Social Services in Northern Ireland. It chairs the Inter-Departmental Working Group on Drugs and Solvents Publicity. It has regular contact with all government departments involved in *Tackling Drugs Together*, including the CDCU. It is represented on the ministerial sub-committee of the Cabinet on the misuse of drugs and on the associated official level committee.

Involvement with other networks

The DoH is involved with: WHO, the UN Drug Control Programme, the Council of Europe's Pompidou Group, the European Union Drug Dependence Unit, and the European Monitoring Centre on Drugs and Drug Addiction.

Doping Control Unit

The Sports Council
Walkden House
3–10 Melton Street
London NW1 2EB
Tel: 0171 383 5667
Fax: 0171 388 1292
e-mail: michelev@cix.compulink.co.uk

For further information contact: Education Information Officer
Range: UK

Services provided

Provides a doping control service to sport and sports organisations. This service has three elements: testing, education and information. Some 10% (growing to 30% over future years) of the unit's budget goes towards drug education and prevention.

Statutory responsibilities

Responsible to the National Heritage department, the UK Sports Council represents the British government on inter-governmental agreements (Memorandum of Understandings), such as the European Convention on Doping in Sport. It was set up by royal charter, which states that it has a responsibility to 'encourage and support the adoption of the highest ethical standards among persons or teams from our United Kingdom participating in sport and physical recreation, and to support or undertake the provision of programmes or facilities for monitoring drug or substance misuse among persons from our United Kingdom participating in sport and physical recreation'.

Funding available

Funding is not available for drug education and prevention activities or projects, though programmes can be supported in other ways. For example, an activity or project with the Sports Council's endorsement can attract funding from commercial sponsors, gain support from sports personalities, or gain access to sporting facilities and equipment.

Links with other agencies

The Doping Control Unit has an advisory group which includes organisational representatives from national drugs agencies. On the Interdepartmental Group on Drugs and Solvents Publicity, it is represented through the Department of National Heritage. It has links with ACPO, the CDCU, and health departments and health education authorities in England, Wales, Scotland and Northern Ireland.

Involvement with other networks

The unit is involved in the ACPO committee on drugs in sport, which produced an educational leaflet on this issue. This committee facilitates links between the DfEE, the DoH, Department of National Heritage, Customs and Excise, and the Local Government Drugs Forum.

Drug Education Forum

National Children's Bureau
8 Wakley Street
London EC1V 7QE
Tel: 0171 843 6000
Fax: 0171 278 9512

For further information contact: Anna Lubelska, Co-ordinator

Services provided

The Drug Education Forum began meeting in November 1994.

The aims of the forum are:

- to bring together a broad range of organisations with a variety of perspectives and develop concerns about drug education issues;
- to provide an independent and authoritative voice for drug education;
- to ensure that it remains a high priority for government and the educational service to encourage the provision of relevant and appropriate drug education for all children and young people;
- to encourage appropriate initial and in-service training for teachers and other professionals involved in providing drug education.

In order to achieve those aims the forum:

- shares and disseminates information and ideas;
- develops agreed criteria for what constitutes effective drug education;
- influences policy makers at different levels to promote the provision of effective drug education;
- stimulates debate about drug education.

Expertise and special knowledge

The forum has over 20 members including: six teaching associations, ACPO, the Drug Education Practitioners Forum, HEA, Hope UK, ISDD, Life Education Centres, NSCoPSE, the National Children's Bureau, the National Health Education Liaison Group, Release, Roehampton Institute, SCODA, and TACADE.

It also has observers from agencies including the CDCU, DfEE, DoH and the Home Office.

Links with other agencies

The forum shares information between its member agencies by circulating papers before and after meetings.

Involvement with other networks

The forum has close links with the Sex Education Forum, which is also based at the National Children's Bureau.

Drug Education Practitioners Forum

c/o Redbridge Drug and Alcohol Service
Gate Cottages
Chadwell Heath Hospital
Romford
Essex RM6 4XJ
Tel: 0181 597 2802
Fax: 0181 503 8718

For further information contact: Sue Cannon, Administrator
Range: UK

Services provided

This is an independent forum for individuals working in drug education, in which they can share information and experience about drug education practice and developments. It is a network of practitioners in drug education, representing a cross section of interests and backgrounds. There are 35 members, of whom between eight and fifteen usually attend meetings.

Its aims are to:

- maintain a high profile for drugs education, by means of contribution to the National Children's Bureau Drug Education Forum and other relevant groups;
- actively explore realistic and effective strategies in drug education;
- show a belief and commitment to the importance of drawing on a wide range of perspectives;
- examine and consider the implications in current research and evaluation findings;
- raise awareness of resources, projects and initiatives;
- provide an opportunity to discuss drug issues;
- help develop effective drug education strategies.

Meetings of the forum are held once a (school) term at the North West London Drugs Prevention Initiative. Particular topics are focused on at each meeting and notes are sent to all members. It has a rotating chairperson.

Membership is £25 to local/health authority/Home Office employees; £12 to consultant or voluntary organisation employees.

Health Education Authority (HEA)

Trevelyan House
30 Great Peter Street
London SW1P 2HW
Tel: 0171 222 5300
Fax: 0171 413 8900

For further information contact: the Drugs Team: Tel. 0171 413 1816

Services provided

The HEA is contracted by the Department of Health to run the drug education and prevention publicity campaign for 11- to 25-year-olds in England. The campaign aims to highlight the health risks associated with the use of illicit drugs and solvents and thereby reduce the acceptability to young people of drug and solvent use. This is part of the government's drugs strategy set out in the White Paper *Tackling Drugs Together*.

The campaign work includes motivating young people to resist drugs through a comprehensive communications programme using an information and 'informed choice' approach. It has included press and radio advertising promoting the National Drugs Helpline and has covered specific drugs such as speed, ecstasy, LSD, magic mushrooms and also mixing drugs. Drugs are covered more generally in leaflets and other promotional materials including new media technology such as the Internet and CD-ROMs. The campaign is underpinned by an extensive 'below the line' press and public relations programme with the youth and adult media.

Support is provided to those who are in contact with young people (parents, teachers, youth workers, health and social workers) through a number of projects, many of which are undertaken in association with other agencies such as ISDD and SCODA. This support element includes needs assessments, regular mailings and updates, provision of resources and information on local education and prevention activity.

The HEA drugs work is informed and developed by a comprehensive research strategy. In addition to the annual survey of 5000 young people which looks at their attitudes, perception and behaviour in relation to drug use, all concepts and campaign materials are tested with target audiences. Focus groups around the country provide an excellent insight into this very fast-moving scene.

The work of the HEA in developing commercial partnerships originated in *Tackling Drugs Together*. Ideal partnerships are those that incorporate activities at both local and national level. The industry sectors particularly targeted are those aimed specifically at young people and parents such as financial institutions, supermarket chains, record stores and clothes shops.

Expertise and special knowledge

Staff have knowledge of health education and promotion principles combined with specialities in fields such as press and publicity, research, and new technology.

Links with other agencies

The drug education publicity campaign has an expert advisory group, which includes representatives from the Home Office DPI, ISDD, Lifeline, the National Addiction Centre, the medical field, SCODA, and social services. Quarterly meetings are held with equivalent drug education departments at the Health Education Board for Scotland, Health Promotion Wales, and the Health Promotion Agency for Northern Ireland. Regular meetings are held and work is also shared with TACADE, Network Scotland, the Local Government Drugs Forum and a range of local and national agencies.

Involvement with other networks

A representative attends the government inter-departmental steering groups on the publicity campaign, and the HEA is a member of the National Children's Bureau Drug Education Forum.

Involvement with local planning

The HEA works with national and local agencies, drug service staff and health professionals in support of the publicity campaign. The HEA also seeks to influence purchasers to make sure health education features in their purchasing plans.

Home Office Drugs Prevention Initiative (DPI)

Central Drugs Prevention Unit

Home Office
Room 354, Horseferry House
Dean Ryle Street
London SW1P 2AW
Tel: 0171 217 8631 (details of local teams available from this number)
Fax: 0171 217 8230

Services provided

The main aim of the Home Office Drugs Prevention Initiative (DPI) is to show clearly what communities can do to prevent drugs misuse. In its second phase, 1995–9, the Home Office DPI has developed a programme of project work, building on its experience since 1990, which explores different approaches to drugs prevention. The programme is being implemented through the DPI's local drugs prevention teams (each comprising five or six staff) which work in partnership with other agencies and organisations in twelve areas in England. The projects, underpinned by a programme of independent research, have been planned to discover what are the most effective approaches and ideas, and in which settings and combinations they produce the most powerful, positive impact on young people's knowledge, attitudes and behaviour towards drugs. The findings will be made available to help people all over the country to take action against drug misuse. Good practice guidance based on earlier work has already been published.

The themes being addressed include:

- community involvement
- work with parents
- young people outside school
- support for drugs education
- peer approaches
- rural communities
- criminal justice
- training for professionals
- local information campaigns
- involvement of racially and culturally diverse groups
- combined approaches
- role of libraries and resource centres.

Statutory responsibilities

The Home Office DPI has no specific statutory responsibilities, but its work contributes directly to the government's drugs strategy set out in the White Paper *Tackling Drugs Together*.

Expertise and special knowledge

Drugs prevention teams include staff with relevant experience from a wide variety of backgrounds. Members of different teams collaborate on the basis of their work in particular parts of the overall programme. With the assistance of administrative staff and specialist research commissioners in the Central Drugs Prevention Unit, and consultancy advice where necessary, these collaborative groups ensure that the work is planned, delivered, monitored and evaluated in ways which provide the best chance of producing valuable findings. This system ensures the maximum use of expertise and experience across the Home Office DPI.

Aside from their work in supporting the national programme, local teams are in a position to offer advice, and sometimes resources, on all aspects of drugs prevention, and especially on consulting and working with communities.

Funding available

Total Home Office DPI grant funding is about £1.9 million per year. The majority of this is committed to the planned programme outlined above, but a proportion is available for teams to support other projects which spring from the agendas of their local communities.

Links with other agencies

Nationally, there is regular consultation between the Home Office DPI and other government departments involved in tackling drug misuse, notably the CDCU, DoH and DfEE. A representative sits on the interdepartmental steering group on publicity, and the Home Office DPI provides evidence and official observers to the Advisory Council on the Misuse of Drugs. There are also links with national drug agencies such as the Institute for the Study of Drug Dependence (ISDD), SCODA, the Advisory Council on Alcohol and Drug Education (TACADE), and educational bodies such as the Roehampton Institute.

Involvement with other networks

Nationally, the Home Office DPI maintains links with bodies such as the Local Government Drugs Forum, the London Drug Policy Forum, the National Children's Bureau Drug Education Forum, and the Drug Education Practitioners Forum.

Involvement in local planning

Drugs prevention teams aim to support and assist the work of local DATs and DRGs. They often sit on these bodies and play an active part in the development of local policies, programmes and plans. They seek to enhance the status of drugs prevention on the agendas of other agencies and to get prevention added to as many agendas as possible.

Hope UK

25f Copperfield Street
London SE1 0EN
Tel: 0171 928 0848
Fax: 0171 401 3477

For further information contact: Martin Perry, National Education Co-ordinator
Range: UK

Services provided

Hope UK is a Christian educational charity. It works with its affiliated groups, members and any other group or individual to reduce alcohol and other drug-related harm in the United Kingdom. With children and young people it aims to achieve this by positive health promotion, including peer-led activities, the promotion of drugfree lifestyles, and the provision of high quality resources and training events.

Links with other agencies

Hope UK is affiliated to the: Charity Forum; English Churches Youth Service; European Blue Cross Youth; Evangelical Alliance; Evangelical Coalition on Drugs; National Council for Voluntary Organisations; National Council for Voluntary Youth Service; National Drug Prevention Alliance (NDPA); Institute of Fundraising Managers; International Blue Cross Federation; Re-Solv; Volunteer Centre (UK).

Institute for the Study of Drug Dependence (ISDD)

Waterbridge House
32–36 Loman Street
London SE1 0EE
Tel: 0171 928 1211
Fax: 0171 928 7071/1771

For further information contact: the Information Service
Range: UK

Services provided

ISDD's objective is to advance knowledge, understanding and policy making about drugs. It is a national provider of drugs information.

Drugs information is:

- generated through consultancy and action research;
- evaluated by reviewing and overviewing existing research;
- disseminated widely, in response to specific requests and via publications.

It has a publicly available library and information service, which is stocked with research published on drug education and prevention. Publications produced to disseminate information gathered include the bi-monthly magazine *Druglink*.

Projects related to drug education and prevention have involved:

- an evaluation of drug education and prevention, including: literature reviews, action research, consultancy and evaluation in schools;
- collaborative work with schools' programmes in Denmark on the medium-term impact of drug education; and on family and community responses to prevention;
- developing mechanisms to deliver information electronically to the education and prevention sector – these include a web site and pages that address questions from the field, and an electronic library service which lists references on education and prevention;
- developing typologies and linguistic equivalences in the field of demand reduction, in collaboration with the European Monitoring Centre on Drugs and Drug Addiction (EMCDDA).

Expertise and special knowledge

ISDD has specialist knowledge of evaluative techniques and methodologies, of different ways of approaching drug education and prevention, of information gathering and dissemination, and of patterns of drug taking behaviour amongst young people.

Links with other agencies

ISDD has funding links with the relevant government departments, including Health, Education, the Home Office, Customs and Excise, and the Foreign Office. It has informal or project-orientated links with other national drugs organisations. ISDD is the operational focal point for EMCDDA, which focuses specifically on drug demand reduction.

Involvement with other networks

ISDD has observers on the National Children's Bureau Drug Education Forum, and links with the National Liaison Group of Co-ordinators of Health and Drugs Education.

Life Education Centres

1st floor, 53–56 Great Sutton Street
London EC1V 0DE
Tel: 0171 490 3210
Fax: 0171 490 3610
e-mail: katnip@lifedn22.demon.co.uk

For further information contact: Michael Roberts, Director
Range: UK

Services provided

Life Education Centres is a charity which provides structured drug prevention and health education programmes for children and young people aged from 3 to 15. The programmes are delivered by highly trained and experienced educators in mobile learning centres which visit schools every year. There are currently 30 Life Education Centres in Britain.

Audio-visuals, an illuminated anatomical model of the human body, electronic modules of the body organs, a talking brain, and Harold, the singing giraffe, are some of the resources in the mobile centre. The trained educator leads the children in learning about the body and how it works, and (for children over eight) about what substances people might use which would change the way the body works, by discussion, role-play, and non-judgemental exploration of the issues surrounding legal and illegal drug use in society.

Publications and follow-up materials are offered to parents, schools and other interested parties to ensure that the programmes are fully integrated into a long-term project.

The aim of the programmes is to provide a community-based resource which will provide children with information and the self-esteem and skills necessary for them to make positive decisions about their own lives, and fulfil their own unique potential.

Expertise and special knowledge

Life Education Centre educators invariably have a teaching degree or background, and relevant experience. They then undergo a rigorous 12-week training course, and thereafter take part in regular workshops. Senior educators and the training officer ensure that programme standards are maintained. Teaching is interactive, child-centred and discussion-based, and uses the resources mentioned to elicit the children's knowledge and attitudes, and to develop these within a safe environment.

Links with other agencies

Life Education has information exchange links with other national drug agencies, and with DATs in the regions where they operate.

Involvement with other networks

Life Education attends meetings of the National Children's Bureau Drug Education Forum. The Director of Research is an observer on the All Party Drugs Misuse Group.

Local Government Drugs Forum (LGDF)

35 Great Smith Street
London SW1P 3BJ
Tel: 0171 222 8100
Fax: 0171 222 0878
e-mail: noel.towe@ama.lgovgs.gov.uk

For further information contact: Noel Towe, Principal Officer
Range: England, Wales and Scotland

Services provided

The LGDF exists to advise and support local authorities in developing drug education and prevention strategies and practical interventions. It lobbies government on behalf of local authority drug interests.

Expertise and special knowledge, and links with other agencies

The forum is structured so that it draws on the expert knowledge in its advisory group. The group consists of 13 councillors, who are nominated by the four local authority associations. It also includes representatives from the DfEE, the HEA, SCODA and TACADE.

Involvement with other networks

It is represented on the National Children's Bureau Drug Education Forum.

Involvement in local planning

LGDF can provide advice to those involved in drug education and prevention at the local level. It has gathered information about local activity, when necessary, for lobbying purposes.

London Drug Policy Forum (LDPF)

Town Clerk's Office
PO Box 270
Guildhall
London EC2P 2EJ
Tel: 0171 332 3084
Fax: 0171 332 3720

For further information contact: Alyson Morley, Policy Adviser
Range: London

Services provided

The LDPF is a London-wide organisation, whose brief is to support and influence 33 London local authorities in their drug policies and practice. The forum consists of elected members from the Association of London Government. It also has an advisory group with representatives from organisations such as apa (Association for the Prevention of Addiction), DfEE, the Home Office, SCODA, London Borough Grants Unit, the Metropolitan Police, health authority representatives, and the Black Drug Workers Forum.

The LDPF's areas of work include:

- community safety (including drug education and prevention in informal settings);
- community care and treatment for drug users;
- drug education and prevention in schools (guidance on policy and practice);
- co-ordinating information on drug education policies and practice across London;
- guidance to licensing authorities and club owners on health and safety at dance events;
- liaison and multi-agency planning of drugs policy and education and prevention.

Expertise and special knowledge

The forum's area of expertise is in providing policy advice on a range of issues including community safety, care and treatment of drug users, education and prevention, and effective multi-agency liaison and planning. To inform its work, it is advised by and works with other specialist agencies.

Links with other agencies

The forum has links with all the London boroughs, health authorities, DATs, the Home Office, SCODA, LGDF, TACADE, the DfEE, CDCU, the Drug Education Forum, the DPI, and the three London Drugs Prevention Teams.

Involvement with other networks

The forum contributes to the LGDF peer education network, and attends the National Children's Bureau Drug Education Forum and a joint Metropolitan Police/National Health Education Liaison Group (NLG) working group.

Involvement in local planning

The forum aims to influence local authorities, and schools, policies and practice with regard to drug-related incidents, education and prevention. It can offer advice and support to local education authorities and schools that are developing policy.

National Drug Prevention Alliance (NDPA)

PO Box 137
London N10 3JJ
Range: UK

Services provided

The NDPA is a network of concerned citizens and prevention professionals who believe that drug-free healthy lifestyles will protect and enhance society and its stability for present and future generations.

NDPA promotes effective policies using all means available to its members, including prevention, education, intervention, treatment, and legal processes.

NDPA resolutions

NDPA will campaign for the potential of prevention approaches to be fulfilled, especially for the very young: a rational and 'seamless' set of policies across all age ranges is the aim; these should ideally combine to form a systematic approach which unites and empowers all sections of society.

Policies and programmes that condone or encourage drug use based on harm reduction are considered unacceptable.

NDPA is in favour of laws which reinforce drug-free and wholly healthy lifestyles, and supports efforts to maintain and improve this situation. It is pressing for improved accurate information and for more accuracy and balance in the media.

Links with other agencies

Through its executive council and its supporters, NDPA links with a wide range of agencies and individuals.

National Health Education Liaison Group (NLG)

Berkshire County Council Education Department
Shire Hall, Shinfield Park
Reading
Berks RG2 9XE
Tel: 01734 234234
Fax: 01734 750360

For further information contact: Adrian King
Range: England and Wales

Services provided

The purpose of the NLG is to promote the entitlement and delivery of quality health education for all young people.

Its aims are:

- to provide personal and professional support to post-holders through regional and national networks;

- to promote health education particularly with regard to alcohol, tobacco and other drugs, and sexual health;
- to act as a network and clearing house for the exchange of related information and ideas;
- to liaise with the Department for Education and Employment (DfEE), other government departments, appropriate parliamentary groups, and other relevant organisations;
- to facilitate co-operative working between post-holders on specific projects and developments.

NLG fulfils its aims by:

- acting as a national and local voice for effective/good practice;
- influencing and affecting national and local policy;
- promoting greater understanding of education for health amongst policy makers, service purchasers and providers;
- providing personal and professional development and support for members.

To do this it engages in:

- information and advice provision;
- liaison with other agencies;
- lobbying and pressure group activity;
- the provision of membership services.

In all its activities NLG:

- upholds equality of opportunity;
- recognises and responds to the needs, views and realities of young people.

It holds:

- national meetings once a (school) term for regional representatives, generally in London;
- a national annual conference at which there is an annual general meeting;
- meetings every six months at the DfEE with the parliamentary under-secretary of state for this area of the school curriculum.

Membership

There are currently 115 members of the group. Membership is open to health education co-ordinators or equivalent whose post has a primary focus of health or drugs education with young people. The annual membership fee is £5.

National Youth Agency (NYA)

17–23 Albion Street
Leicester LE1 6GD
Tel: 0116 285 6789
Fax: 0116 247 1043
e-mail: nya@nyainfo.demon.co.uk

For further information contact: Monica Hingorani, Information Officer

Services provided

The NYA is funded primarily by local authority associations and government departments (DfEE and the Voluntary and Community Division of the Department of National Heritage).

Its communications work includes:

- a series of reading lists on substance misuse, covering the areas of drugs, alcohol, smoking and solvents;
- a briefing paper on *Tackling Drugs Together* with implications for the youth service (1995) which was disseminated to all local authority and national voluntary youth services;
- information support and enquiry answering offered by an information officer with health education as a specialist subject area;
- dissemination of news on national and local initiatives in drug education and prevention work, by means of periodicals such as *Young People Now* and *Policy Update*;
- the production of a training pack for youth workers (1993).

Its initiatives on youth work development include a contract with the DfEE to map and evaluate work funded through GEST 10b (a grant to support training for youth and community workers in raising their awareness of, and developing skills for, dealing with young people at risk from or in the early stages of drug abuse).

Expertise and special knowledge

NYA works with young people on drug education and prevention primarily through the youth and community service.

Funding available

The NYA administers the Youth Work Development Grants on a three-year cycle. In the recent funding cycle, 1995–8, some of these were allocated to organisations running drug education and prevention activities.

Links with other agencies

The NYA has informal links with other agencies that have a role in drug education, including the HEA, ISDD and SCODA. It refers to these agencies for specialist advice.

Involvement with other networks

It is a member of the Adolescent Health Network.

Involvement with local planning

The NYA can support local planning of drug education and prevention by disseminating examples of innovative practice, policy and guidelines through its publications, enquiry service and regional youth work development advisers.

Release   (NVO)

388 Old Street
London EC1V 9LT
Tel: 0171 729 5255
Fax: 0171 729 2599

Range: UK

Services provided

Release provides a range of services dedicated to meeting the health, welfare and legal needs of drug users and those who live and work with them.

These include:

- Drugs in Schools Helpline: offers help and support to pupils, parents and teachers involved in drug related incidents at school;
- media and public policy resource: often called upon to comment on drug related issues which enter the public arena;
- 24-hour telephone helpline: information, advice and support on drugs and legal issues, provided by Release staff and volunteers;
- confidential and professional legal advice about specialist areas of drugs law, as well as general criminal and other procedures for those who come into contact with drugs;
- the Release training programme: operates nationwide offering specialist training on drugs and the law to professionals who work with drug users;
- education and information materials on the legal and health aspects of drug use;
- conferences and events;
- expert evidence at drug trials: providing an unbiased and informed opinion on illicit drug trends, such as current street prices and common methods of drug use.

Standing Conference on Drug Abuse (SCODA)

32–36 Loman Street
London SE1 0EE
Tel: 0171 928 9500
Fax: 0171 928 3343

For further information contact: Steve Taylor, Head of Membership Services
Range: England and Wales

Services provided

SCODA seeks to reduce the harmful effects of drug use through informed debate and the promotion of best practice, and through effective, comprehensive services.

It is an independent membership organisation, providing a voice for drug services and others concerned about the effects of drug use on individuals and communities.

SCODA is developing its work in drug education and prevention. It works for those developing, providing and purchasing in this field by:

- influencing national policy and providing information services and publications;
- operating an education and prevention information exchange on innovation, standards, and good practice in service delivery;
- supporting training, quality assurance and accreditation for drug education and prevention services.

Statutory responsibilities

SCODA's role as identified by the White Paper *Tackling Drugs Together* is to:

- represent service providers accross the spectrum of education, prevention, treatment and care;
- provide advice to members on standards, quality of care and value for money;
- accredit members who deliver those standards;
- disseminate good practice to providers;
- give information on training to providers;
- give advice to the government on emerging trends in substance misuse;
- advise the government on innovative primary and secondary prevention which might benefit from 'seed corn' funding;
- consider what more can be done to increase the safety of communities and reduce the susceptibility of young people to drug misuse.

Expertise and special knowledge

SCODA is a focal point for contact information on drug services (including education and prevention, treatment, care and rehabilitation) in England and Wales.

In supporting drug services, it draws on its staff expertise in information technology and systems, training and accreditation, research and evaluation, grants administration and project management.

Funding available

SCODA administered the DoH's Young People at Risk of Drugs grants scheme in 1995–6, and the Esmée Fairbairn Charitable Trust small grants schemes in 1995 and 1996.

Links with other agencies

SCODA is represented on the HEA's expert advisory group. With ISDD it jointly provides the secretariat to the All Party Drugs Misuse Group. Chief Executive, Roger Howard, sits on the Advisory Council on the Misuse of Drugs.

SCODA also co-ordinates and services a number of specialist forums including:

- the Drug Policy Forum;
- the Drug Training and Development Forum.

Involvement with other networks

SCODA is a member of the National Children's Bureau Drug Education Forum.

TACADE
(The Advisory Council on Alcohol and Drug Education)

1 Hulme Place
The Crescent, Salford
Manchester M5 4QA
Tel: 0161 745 8925
Fax: 0161 745 8923
e-mail: tacade@dial.pipex.com

For further information contact: Mandy Broadbent, Head of Projects and Marketing
Range: UK

Services provided

TACADE is a national non-government organisation specialising in personal, social and health education.

It aims to provide a service for professional groups, parents and carers in the promotion of healthy lifestyles and behaviour, and the prevention of drug misuse. It has three main areas of work in drug education and prevention:

- development and production of resource material;
- training provision and conference administration;
- project development, management and consultancy.

TACADE's work is targeted at all sectors of the population, but has particular reference to the needs of young people and those who care, and have responsibility, for them.

Current TACADE projects include:

- Alcohol Education in the Primary School;
- Skills for Life evaluation;
- Health Promoting Primary Schools;
- Drug Education for Parents;
- review of materials for training in research and evaluation skills;
- working in Northern Ireland to increase its activity and support for drug education and prevention initiatives;
- Acting for Health;
- animation;
- development of a handbook for sports coaches and teachers on the topic of drugs in sport;
- Learning for Life;
- Iceland Frozen Foods Drug Prevention in Schools Initiative;
- training courses for teachers with the Cheshire Partnership.

Recently completed projects include:

- implementation of drug education in Europe;
- *Fit for football* (a drug education leaflet);
- drug education for offenders.

Expertise and special knowledge

TACADE has particular expertise and experience in drug misuse prevention and intervention. Its staff includes a qualified team of professional trainers and consultants, who have experience and expertise in health, education, research, training, nursing, and administration. Staff have all been actively involved in the research, development and writing of numerous resource materials.

Links with other agencies

TACADE staff are currently members of, or affiliated to, the following groups: Advisory Council on the Misuse of Drugs, Prevention Working Party; Addictions Forum; LGDF; ACPO Working Party on Partnerships in Drug Misuse; National Children's Bureau Drug Education Forum; and SCODA.

TACADE provides consultancy to individual schools on the review, development and implementation of health, personal, and social education and lifeskills education.

It also has international and European affiliations, and staff work as consultants to the European Commission, the United Nations Drug Control Programme, the World Health Organization and UNICEF. It is partner to the Global Initiative on Primary Prevention of Substance Abuse.

Involvement with other networks

TACADE seeks to work with a wide variety of groups and organisations including: schools, the National Health Service, the police, the probation service, alcohol and drugs agencies, charitable organisations, the youth service, Home Office Drug Prevention Teams, national and local service organisations, national and local government, training organisations, industry, and international agencies.

Involvement in local planning

TACADE is not involved in drug education and prevention at a strategic planning level, but aims to work with and support local agencies in the statutory and non-statutory sector, particularly local education authorities and Health Promotion Units.

Directory of local organisations and activities

General notes to the directory section

This Directory contains entries for organisations by county. Within each county entries are arranged alphabetically by town and then by organisation. Activities are listed alphabetically after their associated organisation.

Organisation entries

It has been assumed throughout that drugs work is the 'main business' of an organisation unless otherwise stated. Where an organisation provides 'other drug services' (in addition to drug education and/or prevention) these are shown.

Activity entries

Specific target groups are only given where appropriate and where these have not been made clear in the description of an activity.

Contents

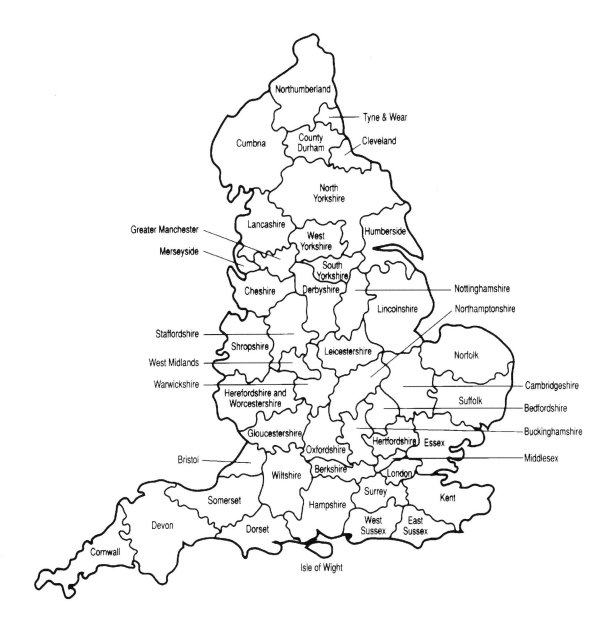

Map of England showing geographical boundaries

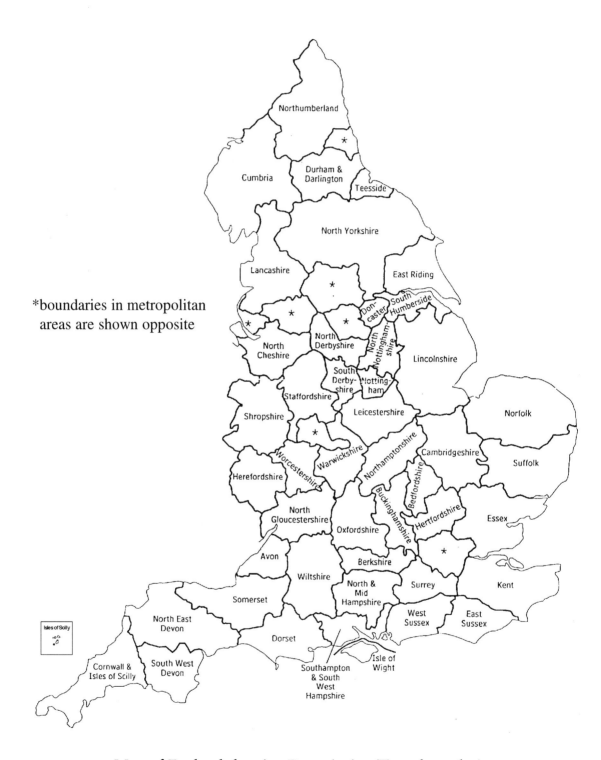

*boundaries in metropolitan areas are shown opposite

Map of England showing Drug Action Team boundaries

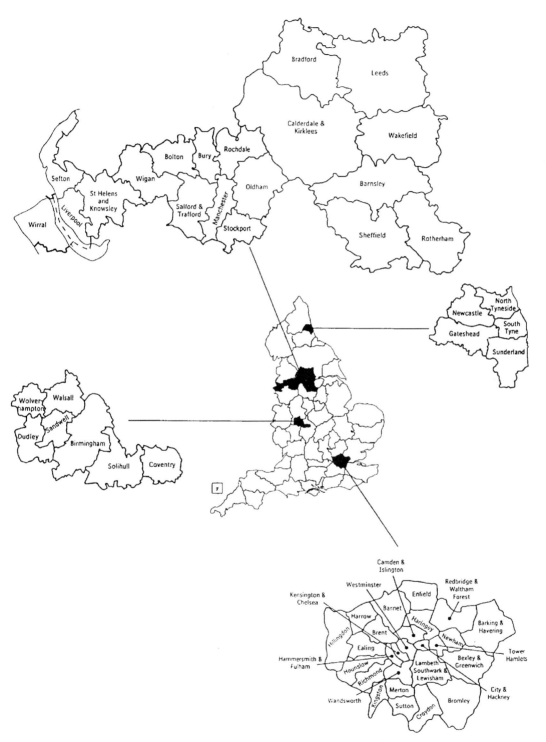

Drug Action Team boundaries in metropolitan areas

Bedfordshire

PLAN-B: PEER-LED ACTION NETWORK – BEDFORD

26 Bromham Road, Bedford MK40 2QD

Tel: 01234 270123

Contact: Sue Reed

Health authority: Bedfordshire

Other drug services: Treatment; training

Peer training

This is a training programme for 14–20-year-olds to enable them to talk with peer groups about drugs. The project also involves supporting this work and developing community links.

Contact: Sue Reed

Tel: 01234 270123

Partners: Health Authority; education; youth service; charities

Funder: Department of Health

Needs assessment methods: A questionnaire was sent out on drug use among young people and what they perceived as service needs.

Target age groups: 14–20

Target groups: Offenders; not at school; children in care

Methods and evaluation: The programme includes a training package for self-selecting groups of volunteers as well as back-up for peer trainers in planning, delivering and evaluating the service.

Training is evaluated by trainees and through modified, written, and scaled evaluation sheets. Independent evaluation is through monitoring activity and analysing outcomes.

RED HERRING PRODUCTIONS

SFK Technology Ltd, Cranfield, Bedford MK43 OAJ

Tel: 01234 752295   **Fax:** 01234 752305

Contact: Linton Bocock

Health authority: Bedfordshire

Main business: The development of innovative projects which seek to further the good of the community in terms of health and well-being

Sharing the Message

The project is aimed at upper schools and youth groups in the North Bedfordshire area. The aim of the project is to explore the issues surrounding substance misuse from the perspective of a creative writer. The resulting ideas are then presented in a dramatic format.

Contact: Linton Bocock

Tel: 01234 270123

Partners: Health Link; Drugs and Alcohol Advisory Service

Funders: European Drug Prevention Week; Eastern Arts Board, Bedfordshire County Council Health Link

Target age groups: 11–21

Methods and evaluation: Session 1: Participants critically assess TV adverts and public information films for their ability to effectively communicate. Session 2: Participants take part in a fact-finding exercise designed to inform them about six popular drugs. Sessions 3 and 4: Participants conceive and develop ideas concerning substance misuse. These ideas are aimed at a chosen target group. Session 5: Presentation of pieces to class, followed by a critical assessment of each piece. Follow-up: A written assessment in questionnaire format.

The participants and teacher/group leaders complete questionnaires. The project leader combines these in a project report.

SANDY YOUTH CLUB

Park Road, Sandy, Bedfordshire SG19 1JB

Tel: 01767 680583

Contact: D Ploszay

Health authority: Bedfordshire

Other drug services: Training

Main business: Youth work

Peer health education group

The initiative aims to establish a group of young peer educators who will prevent other young people from starting to use drugs.

Contact: D Ploszay

Tel: 01767 680583

Funder: County youth service

Target age group: 11–16

Methods: A group of four young people have committed themselves to a further 20 hours of training in peer education. It is intended to produce leaflets, posters and quizzes, etc., and to visit voluntary and statutory youth clubs in the area in order to give information on the dangers of drug misuse, practice in saying 'no', and to hold group discussions.

Berkshire

PPP (POSITIVE PREVENTION PLUS)

3 Radnor Way, Slough, Berkshire SL3 7LA

Tel: 01753 542296   **Fax:** 01753 542296

Contacts: Peter Stoker/Ann Stoker

Health authority: Berkshire

Other drug services: Treatment; community safety; training; consultancy, policy, leaflets, exhibitions; media work; referrals

Parenting Skills for Prevention

This is an initiative to develop competency and confidence in parents trying to get their children drug free from adolescence to adulthood, and to bring parents back from the margins.

Contacts: Peter Stoker, Ann Stoker

Tel: 01753 542296

Funder: Self-funded; evaluation funded by Home Office Drug Prevention Initiative

Needs assessment methods: A university-based literature study (international) was completed, with observations in street drug agency, drug dependency advice centre, and community settings. There was a clear need for skilling/strengthening parents.

Target groups: Parents and grandparents

Methods and evaluation: The project is based on the PRIDE 'Parent to Parent' video/audio-based programme, written by a former youth rehab director now specialising in prevention (see *Drug prevention – first day now* by Peter Stoker (1992), pages 67–72). The project takes place through exhibitions and presentations, and occasionally in workplaces. Peter and Ann Stoker were trained/accredited in the USA.

Evaluation is by participants, staff, an independent evaluator (education specialist), and the funder.

Participants and volunteers give exit evaluations. These include independent evaluations; literature study; vetting other evaluations; in-depth interviews; comparison with experience.

TEENEX

This is an experiential learning project with a high-peer education component aimed at producing peer leaders/educators. The main vehicle is a one-week lock-in with a busy curriculum.

Contacts: Dave Perry, Roger Hill

Tel: 01702 558820

Funders: Self-funded; police; Glaxo; minor donations

Needs assessment methods: A review of youth drug prevention was carried out as well as an international literature search of prevention needs/responses.

Target age groups: 11 and over

Target group: Parents

Methods and evaluation: The project uses exhibitions, presentations and camps.

The projects are currently under evaluation in Germany, and have been evaluated in Poland and Portugal.

Evaluation is by participants/staff through exit evaluations and one three-year retro. In addition there have been evaluations by the following: an independent (UK); St John's Ambulance; Essex Police in 1993/4, who reviewed all papers/ evaluations to date and observed operations.

Bristol

BADMINTON ROAD METHODIST YOUTH CENTRE

Badminton Road, Downend, Bristol BS16 6NU

Tel: 0117 956 3833

Contact: Maggie Curtis

Health authority: Avon

Main business: Working with young people in the area of Downend, Bristol

Positive Risk Taking

This initiative encourages young people, through education and positive risk taking, to seek alternatives to drug use, to stop using drugs and to reduce harm to those who are using drugs.

Contact: Maggie Curtis

Tel: 0117 956 3833

Funders: Methodist church, local authority

Methods and evaluation: The activity takes place in the Fedw activity centre in the Brecon Beacons with specific exercises, i.e. use of substance identification cards, questionnaires, graffiti boards and games; education through use of videos, posters, and leaflets; education through physical activity, i.e. climbing, go-karting, canoeing, caving, etc; and education through residential experiences – living logistics, negotiating, sharing, and good role models.

Evaluation was carried out through discussion with young people and staff during funding from Young People at Risk from Drugs, and regular end-of-evening meetings.

A report was written and sent to the Innovations Group about a project funded through Young People at Risk from Drugs (DoH grant scheme).

CRISIS CENTRE MINISTRIES

12 City Road, St Pauls, Bristol BS2 8TP

Tel: 0117 942 3088   **Fax:** 0117 924 0799

Contact: Derek Groves

Health authority: Avon

Other drug services: Treatment; training; drop-in weekly support group

Bus Stop Project

The project aims to provide a mobile centre for outreach to young people on the streets and in the community who are involved in drugs/alcohol.

Contact: Derek Groves

Tel: 0117 942 3088

Partner: The Muller Foundation

Funder: Crisis Centre Ministries

Needs assessment methods: The assessment was undertaken by the Muller Foundation.

Target age groups: 11–21

Target groups: Homeless; parents

Methods and evaluation: Jointly with the Muller Foundation, the project provides a mobile centre as a point of contact where young people are already congregating. It is presently establishing relationships with a view to offering education, advice, etc.

The Missing Peace

This is a drop-in centre for people with life-controlling difficulties.

Contact: Derek Groves

Tel: 0117 9423088

Funders: Crisis Centre Ministries

Target age groups: 17 and over

Target groups: Offenders; homeless; neighbourhoods

Methods and evaluation: The drop-in centre is a non-threatening place to meet, offering low-price meals and a meal-voucher scheme. It provides counselling, information, referral to rehab, etc.

An outside body completed a detailed audit of the work. A management council regularly reviews progress and the director evaluates the effectiveness of the approach.

DAC (DRUGS AWARENESS CAMPAIGN)

PO Box 565, Bristol BS99 5YZ

Tel: 0117 951 1556   **Fax:** 0117 951 1556

Contact: Tony Hall

Health authority: Avon

Other drug services: Criminal justice; training; temporary jobs

Main business: Raising funds to increase awareness of the problems of drugs misuse

Drug-free events

These events are targeted at the 8–16-year-olds, and aim to give credibility to drug-free entertainment within the current youth culture.

Contact: Devon Morgan

Tel: 0117 951 1556

Partners: Shoc Wave Records; D&M Media Services; Fresh Nation

Funder: DAC membership

Needs assessment methods: Market research was carried out to assess the need.

Target age group: 8–16

Target groups: Offenders; neighbourhoods

DRUGS AND YOUNG PEOPLE PROJECT

Tyndall's Centre, Southmead Hospital, Westbury on Trym, Bristol BS10 5NB

Tel: 0117 959 5033 **Fax:** 0117 959 5031

Contact: Paul Matthews

Health authority: Avon

Other drug services: Community care, assessment, contracting

Main business: HIV/AIDS and sex industry workers support

Drugs and Young People Project

This project involves early intervention work with clients of Bristol social services (18 years and under). One project worker purchases direct services and provides an operational and consultation role to staff and for training.

Contact: Paul Matthews

Tel: 0117 959 5033

Partners: Social Services; health; freelance counsellors; youth services

Funders: Health Authority; Social Services

Needs assessment methods: A survey of drug use among Social Services department's clients led to an application for funding to Young People at Risk from Drugs (DoH grant scheme). Needs were established through contact with Social Services staff. The training needs assessment is ongoing.

Target age groups: 11–18

Target groups: Offenders; not at school; children in care; Social Services' clients

Methods and evaluation: Detached youth workers engage drug-using clients in various activities. The project provides counselling, group work and leaflets; and trains generic staff in basic drugs education techniques.

Evaluation is by an independent body, Lucas and Sandberg, using meetings, targets and milestones, which are shown to staff. Training evaluation includes experimental design using control and experimental groups to assess the effectiveness of the work.

KINGSWOOD BUS PROJECT

Badminton Road Youth Centre, Badminton Road, Downend, Bristol BS16 6NU

Tel: 0117 956 3833

Contact: June Yeoman

Health authority: Avon

Kingswood Bus Project

The project works with young people who meet on the streets, and as it is mobile, it can work with young people in areas with very few resources. The project aims to achieve: greater awareness by young people of drug and alcohol use; a resource base for young people, staff and volunteers, providing accurate information on drugs and alcohol; and an environment where young people can openly discuss their experiences of drug and alcohol use.

Contact: June Yeoman

Tel: 0117 956 3833

Partners: Police; Health Authority; councils

Funders: South Gloucestershire Council, crime prevention; grants; trusts; charities; local businesses

Needs assessment methods: After the research was funded, it was decided that a mobile resource would be the most effective way of working with large groups of young people on the streets.

Target age groups: 11–21

Target group: Neighbourhoods

Methods and evaluation: The project uses a wide range of materials and resources, from both national and local agencies, in a fun way and in an unusual environment. Relationships are developed with young people in the community and in schools and they are encouraged to talk about drug use/misuse. There is a variety of choices open to young people to enable them to take greater control of their lives.

Evaluation is usually carried out through a questionnaire at the beginning and end. Regular meetings enable staff to discuss the work.

KNOWLE WEST NEIGHBOURHOOD DETACHED PROJECT

Filwood Social Centre, Barnstaple Road, Knowle West, Bristol BS4 1JP

Tel: 0117 953 3290

Contacts: Mike Buckland, Jill James

Health authority: Avon

Main business: Outreach

Knowle West Detached Project

This project works with young people who choose not to use any of the current youth work and provisions. It offers advice and support on contraception, drugs and housing, acting as an advocate for young people and as a referral point for other agencies.

Contact: Mike Buckland

Tel: 0117 953 3290

Funders: Bristol Leisure Services; Single Regeneration Budget 1 and 2; Social Services

Target groups: Offenders; not at school; homeless; neighbourhoods

Methods: The aim is to provide harm minimisation education and safer sex practice, and to try and address the issues that face young people in the area. The project provides young people with relevant literature and a full range of contraception, and also acts as an advocate in courts, at case conferences, and wherever young people need support.

WESTERN ALCOHOL AND DRUGS EDUCATION SOCIETY (WADES)

6 Gloucester Street, Upper Eastville, Bristol BS5 6QE

Tel: 0117 951 2187

Contact: Reverend R Foster

Health authority: Avon

Drugs education delivery

This initiative provides professional personnel to work in schools, churches and secular organisations. It exhibits current educational material relating to all drugs in various venues, including public libraries.

Contact: Sue Thorne

Tel: 0117 951 2187

Funders: Churches; members' subscriptions and donations

Methods: Individual programmes are compiled and executed on the basis of needs, age, background, etc. of the group concerned, in consultation with the group leader. Relevant resources are used, depending on what is required and appropriate.

Buckinghamshire

CHILTERN YOUTH CENTRE

Chiltern Avenue, Amersham, Buckinghamshire HP6 5AH

Tel: 01494 725630

Contact: Ann Stone

Health authority: Buckinghamshire

Other drug services: Treatment; training

Main business: Supporting personal development of young people

Dance Drama Production

This is a peer education project using dance/drama skills.

Contact: Ann Stone

Tel: 01494 725630

Funder: Chiltern Youth Centre

Target age group: 11–16

Methods and evaluation: Young people develop their own awareness of and attitude to drugs, with a staff support plan. Then they organise and create a dance/drama production based on a young woman's involvement with drugs and the consequences. They are also involved in designing and making scenery and costumes.

Evaluation is by a preview shown to an invited audience and feedback/discussion afterwards.

Poster design

Young people design a poster on drugs education to appeal to their peers.

Contact: Ann Stone

Tel: 01494 725630

Funder: Chiltern Youth Centre

Target age groups: 11–16

Methods and evaluation: The group engage in discussion with staff to develop their knowledge of drugs and examine their own attitudes and feelings. Young people then use their ideas and thoughts to develop and design posters appropriate to their own age group.

Evaluation is through discussion on the process of work, design and use of the poster.

Cambridgeshire

CAMBRIDGESHIRE LOCAL EDUCATION AUTHORITY

C105 Castle Court, Shire Hall, Castle Hill, Cambridge CB3 0AP

Tel: 01223 317459   **Fax:** 01223 318180

Contact: Jon Pratt

Health authority: Cambridgeshire

Main business: Education and support

Big Chill Over Cambridgeshire

Activities centre on a training and support theatre-in-education experience for young people for whom school may not be the preferred learning venue. The project runs until August 1997.

Contact: Ruth Joyce

Tel: 01223 317459

Partners: Drug agencies; youth and community service; Social Services; community police

Funders: Local Education Authority, private local funds

Needs assessment methods: Discussions were held with youth and community tutors, young people, Social Services and drug agencies.

Target age group: 11–16

Target groups: Not at school; children in care; neighbourhoods; rural communities

Methods and evaluation: The project provides youth work training on the use of theatre and on drugs awareness. A theatre piece is developed by and with young people, and workshops are followed up, including a discussion with drug agencies.

Parent Awareness Programme

The programme develops parents' awareness of the drugs young people may have contact with, and provides strategies for prevention and for management of drug misuse, as well as help and support.

Contact: Roger Daw

Tel: 01223 317459

Partners: Drug agencies; alcohol agencies; community police

Funders: Locally raised funds

Needs assessment methods: Head teachers' meetings were held.

Target group: Parents

Methods: Meetings are held in the evenings for parents, with participation by representatives of a local drug agency, the police, etc., to encourage multi-agency focus. Written information is provided.

DIAL DRUGLINK

Whitwell Chambers, Ferrars Road, Huntingdon, Cambridgeshire PE18 6DH

Tel: 01480 413800   **Fax:** 01480 411914

Contact: Verina McEwen

Health authority: Cambridgeshire

Other drug services: Treatment; training

Dial Druglink drop-in

The drop-in provides a safe environment to talk about issues and concerns.

Contact: Julie Minney

Tel: 01480 413800

Funder: Cambridgeshire and Huntingdon Health Authority

Needs assessment methods: this was by client feedback.

Target groups: Offenders; homeless; children in care; rural communities

Grants for Education Support and Training (GEST) 19C

This is a theatre-in-education programme that takes place throughout the county.

Contact: Sheilla Duggan

Tel: 01480 413800

Partners: Local Education Authority; drug agencies; community education; police; Social Services

Funders: Department for Education and Employment; local businesses

Target age groups: 11–18

Target groups: Offenders; not at school; children in care

County Durham

DARLINGTON YOUTH DEVELOPMENT TRUST

Haughton Youth Centre, Rockwell Avenue, Darlington, County Durham DL1 2AX

Tel: 01325 380747

Contact: Sue Davidson

Health authority: South Durham

Other drug services: Training

Main business: Social and personal development of young people within the Darlington area

Drug Awareness Project

The project aim is to develop a peer support network for young people at risk from drugs. A total of 24 young people, who were either already involved, or at risk from becoming involved, with drugs were selected to undertake training to eventually form peer support. The project ran until February 1996.

Contact: Sue Davidson

Tel: 01325 380747

Partners: South Durham Community Education Service; Elmfield Centre; Health Authority (young persons' clinic)

Funders: Young People at Risk from Drugs (DoH grant scheme); community education

Needs assessment methods: The following assessments were carried out: a research study,

Two cultures, September 1993; Darlington Borough Council social audit, 1995; and face-to-face contact with detached youth workers.

Target age groups: 11–18

Methods and evaluation: Young people, referred by detached youth workers, may attend a one-week residential course – a combination of outdoor activities and discussions; a workshop – held at eight local venues; or a one-week residential course – a combination of outdoor activities and discussions. Young people deliver drug education sessions in schools and youth centres using material they have developed.

Evaluation is through: Young People at Risk from Drugs Project Milestones, and questionnaires.

Teen Spirit – the video

The project seeks to demystify some health services for young people and to show how helpful and approachable they can be. Focusing on the young people's clinic (contraception, etc.), the Elmfield Centre (addiction service), and the GUM clinic (sexual health treatment centre), young people take a light-hearted look at how to access the services.

Contact: Sue Davidson

Tel: 01325 380247

Partners: Community education (South Durham); South Durham Health Authority

Funders: Regional health authority grant; community education

Target age groups: 11–18

Methods and evaluation: Young people with a specific interest in drama are invited to produce a video demystifying services and showing how easy it is to access them. The young people decide on the content and produce a script. Specialist workers (drama and video makers), work with the young people to produce the video, as the basis for a training package to be used in local schools and youth centres. A credit-card-sized information leaflet with details of agencies will be distributed as part of the training package.

Evaluation is to be based on the numbers of young people taking up the training package, any increase in numbers accessing services, and evaluation sheets for young people taking training.

Derbyshire

CASTLE DONINGTON DRUGS EDUCATION PROJECT

Castle Donington College, Mount Pleasant, Castle Donington, Derbyshire DE74 2LN

Tel: 01332 810528

Contact: Jill Carter

Health authority: Leicestershire

Castle Donington Drugs Education Project

The project aims: to increase young people's drugs awareness/knowledge, to enable them to take the lead in promoting drugs prevention amongst their peers; to enhance the relationship between young people and their community; and to raise the profile of, and instigate action about, issues facing young people in a rural community.

Contact: Jill Carter

Tel: 01332 810528

Partners: District Council; parish council; Turning Point; police; Local Education Authority; local community

Funders: East Midlands Drug Prevention Team; Local Education Authority, youth and community education

Target age groups: 11–21

Target groups: Users of amphetamines, cannabis, ecstasy; parents; neighbourhoods; community groups; rural communities; local villages

Evaluation: Evaluation is by the local community/police. This project is part of the Drugs Prevention Initiative programme of work and is being formally researched via the following: regular meetings between Jill Carter and East Midlands Drug Prevention Team; use of standard data collection instruments devised by the Drugs Prevention Initiative; informal written and verbal feedback to Jill Carter, e.g. press coverage, reports, minutes of meetings, and evaluation sheets.

THE PHOENIX PROJECT

Rosehill Business Centre, Normanton Road, Derby DE23 6RH

Tel: 01332 294 898   **Fax:** 01332 299156

Contact: Leona Stanley

Health authority: South Derbyshire

Other drug services: Community safety; health promotion; information and advice

Main business: Health promotion; sexual health and drugs

David Plackett Dance Drugs Project

This project involves: working with young people on their own territory to help them become better informed about dance drugs; and working with nightclub staff to provide a safer environment. It has also drawn up the criteria on which licensing would ultimately hinge: running drinking water, 'cooling off' areas, first aid, etc.

Contact: David Finn

Tel: 01332 340251

Partners: Derby City Council Youth Service; South Derby Health Authority; Health Promotion Unit; Derby City Council Environmental Health

Funders: Young People at Risk from Drugs (DoH grant scheme); Derby Drugline

Needs assessment methods: Pilot visits to clubs, observations, talks with drug squad and environmental health revealed that water was being turned off in clubs; clubs did have drugs in them; and there were no facilities for chilling out or first aid.

Target age groups: 11 and over

Target groups: Users of dance drugs; neighbourhoods; dance clubs

Methods and evaluation: A total of 10 workers in four clubs engaged young people and staff, giving information and advice where appropriate, e.g. drug usage services available, safer practices, and harm minimisation. They provided support and, where necessary, referrals to other agencies (ambulances, etc.) and occasional first aid. They contributed to the formulation of worker protocol and a code of ethics, and also carried out work in pubs/central areas/streets, and trained other workers.

Evaluation is by Young People at Risk from Drugs, through use of reports, questionnaires involving participants, and tape recordings.

Frontline Peer Education Drug Project

During the project, 15 African Caribbean and Asian volunteers are put through a programme of drug training (delivered from a black perspective) which equips them to deliver drug education to other young black people.

Contact: Leona Stanley

Tel: 01332 294898

Partners: Nottingham Black Initiative; Leicestershire Community Drug Services

Funders: Home Office Drug Prevention Initiative; Southern Derbyshire Health; Derby Pride

Needs assessment methods: Consultation with African Caribbean and Asian young people revealed that peer pressure was a major influence in their lives.

Target age groups: 11 and over

Target groups: Black Caribbean; black African; black other; Indian; Pakistani; Bangladeshi

Methods: The peer educators deliver anti-drug and safer use messages to young people in schools, colleges, youth projects, raves, nightclubs and on the street. Conventional methods of drug education are inappropriate to the needs of black people, who are often portrayed as users or dealers. This project takes a non-Eurocentric perspective to drug education and is delivered by people who understand the experience of other young black people.

Streetwise Education

This initiative aims to work with primary and secondary schools and youth clubs to develop policy and practice on drug education which addresses issues for black comunities.

Contact: Leona Stanley

Tel: 01332 294898

Partner: Derbyshire Education Service

Funder: Home Office Drug Prevention Initiative

Needs assessment methods: Consultation with young black people identified the inappropriateness of the drug education being received.

Target age groups: 11 and over

Target groups: Black Caribbean; black African; black other; Indian; Pakistani; Bangladeshi

Methods: The focus of this project is to work with teachers and youth workers to improve their knowledge and skills when working with young black people. The project also engages young people themselves to develop resources and other projects that involve the local community on drugs prevention activities.

PEER YOUTH INFORMATION ADVICE SERVICE

Community Education Office, Highfields School, Lumsdale Road, Matlock, Derbyshire DE4 5NA

Tel: 01629 584336   **Fax:** 01629 57572

Contact: Jennie Merriman

Health authority: North Derbyshire

Other drug services: Community safety

Main business: Advice and information for young people covering all issues

Peer youth information and advice service

This service is based on peer advice and information workers – volunteers whose natural capacity and willingness to help others has been developed through appropriate training and supervision to provide listening skills and support to their peers in schools and youth club settings.

Contact: Jennie Merriman

Tel: 01629 584336

Partners: Youth service; social work; Social Services; Local Education Authority; police; volunteers

Funders: Youth service; Social Services, Local Education Authority

Needs assessment methods: A survey of 480 young people found that 96 per cent thought it important to have an information/advice service over a range of issues, with drugs and alcohol being very high on the agenda. In addition, 76 per cent said they would use the service.

Target age groups: 11–18

Target group: Rural communities

Methods: Young people produce their own information and publicity and develop their own resource library. As this is a new project, the pro-active side will be negotiated with young people during the training programme, depending on their skills, to be run over the summer holidays.

DERBYSHIRE CONSTABULARY

Police Headquarters, Butterly Hall, Ripley, Derbyshire DE21 5BP

Tel: 01773 572217   **Fax:** 01773 572029

Contact: Inspector Tony Harper

Health authority: North Derbyshire

Other drug services: Community safety; criminal justice

Main business: Producing leaflets on truancy and bullying

Outreach

Outreach activities aim: to prevent young people from starting to use drugs; to encourage young people who use drugs to stop using drugs; and to minimise harm to young drug users.

Contact: Constable Casswell

Tel: 01773 522026

Partner: HM Prison Sudbury, Derbyshire

Funders: Police; Ilkeston Consumer Co-op; Heanor Rotary Club

Target groups: not at school; children in care; parents; community groups

Evaluation: This is through feedback forms.

Devon

THE YOUTH TRUST

The Inn, 6 Market Street, Barnstaple, Devon EX31 1BX

Tel: 01271 321100   **Fax:** 01271 321200   **e-mail:** 101352,466@compuserve.com

Contact: William Palin

Health authority: North and East Devon

The Inn Project

This project aims to provide a credible, sophisticated alternative to illegal drug experimentation for 13–25-year-olds. It incorporates a coffee bar (13–17-year-olds) run by young people, and training facilities, including peer education.

Contact: Will Palin

Tel: 01271 321100

Partners: North Devon District Council; The Quay Centre; youth justice; probation service; East and North Devon Health Authority; Devon Consortium Partnership

Funders: North Devon District Council; various

Needs assessment methods: A study carried out in consultation with the local drug rehabilitation centre and other agencies identified £22.5 million of drug-related crime annually in north Devon.

Target age groups: 13–25

Target groups: Parents; rural communities

Methods: The project provides a social centre specifically for 13–17-year-olds who are most at risk from drug dealers in the district.

EXETER DRUGS PROJECT

Dean Clarke House, Southernhay East, Exeter, Devon EX1 1PQ

Tel: 01392 410292   **Fax:** 01392 499458

Contact: Kim Hager

Health authority: North and East Devon

Other drug services: Treatment; community safety; criminal justice; training

Detached services for young people

The services aim to target young people who: don't use drugs; are on the brink/dabbling; or are involved in regular recreational use. It also assists other staff in contact with young people to work with young people and drugs.

Contact: Kim Hager

Tel: 01392 410292

Funders: Young People at Risk from Drugs (DoH grant scheme); Devon Care Trust

Target age groups: 11 and over

Target groups: Not at school; children in care

Methods: The services offer: tasks, training events, first-aid training, theatre-in-education, peer education, and training of ex-users and dabblers to teach others, working alongside detached workers. Specific literature is aimed at young people. In addition they offer: mobile phone lines; drop-in sessions in local areas; life skills teaching; a quiz on the streets with young people which led to setting up venues in the evening with workshops, disc jockeying, etc; working with local communities, when problems arise, to develop local responses; and expertise and support for police, youth justice team, residential care homes, etc.

HARBOUR CENTRE ALCOHOL AND DRUGS ADVISORY SERVICE

9–10 Ermington Terrace, Mutley, Plymouth, Devon PL4 6QG

Tel: 01752 228986   **Fax:** 01752 256979

Health authority: South and West Devon

Other drug services: Treatment; community safety; criminal justice; training

Main business: Alcohol and drugs agency

Community harm reduction

The project provides community-based support around substance issues linked to relevant agencies, networking as much support as possible, raising awareness, and enabling people to make informed choices to help reduce substance-related risks.

Tel: 01752 228986

Partners: Community groups; health services; police; probation; Social Services; parents

Funder: Health Authority

Needs assessment methods: Community workers used their networks to go through guided questions. Participants met and had the feedback presented to them. Work was then developed and a strategy negotiated.

Target groups: Offenders; not at school; homeless; children in care; parents; neighbourhoods; community groups; rural communities

Methods and evaluation: The project draws on various approaches dependent on need, circumstances and resources. Many people leave with information packs, and then become an information resource in their own street/locality/agency, etc.

Evaluation is qualitative and quantitive. Each participant goes through an evaluation in which the key parts reflect how they felt personally and how they felt they could help their community. An independent institution is looking to evaluate the work from now on.

MDA (MORE DRUGS AWARENESS) – PEER EDUCATION PROJECT

81 Clifton Place, Greenbank, Plymouth, Devon PL1 8HY

Tel: 01752 222627

Contact: Vicky Brooks

Health authority: South and West Devon

MDA peer education project

The project aims to raise awareness and provide accurate and unbiased information about drug-related issues in order to enable young people across Devon to make informed choices and minimise the harm associated with drug use. The project ended in June 1996, and its future depends on further funding.

Contact: Vicky Brooks

Tel: 01752 222627

Partners: Devon Consortium; Health Authority; police; community education

Funders: Young People at Risk from Drugs (DoH grant scheme); Health Authority, County Council

Target age groups: 11 and over

Target groups: Rural communities; youth settings outside school

Methods and evaluation: The peer educators work in groups of two or more with young people on their own territory. They aim to create a safe, relaxed environment where young people feel able to contribute to and discuss drug-related issues. This is achieved by means of fun, participative games and exercises which explore existing knowledge, build upon it by raising awareness and examining attitudes, and promote discussion in a relaxed, non-threatening manner. Exercises are also used which explore and promote life skills such as assertiveness. Examples of exercises used are: brainstorming; case studies; role-plays; guided discussion; interactive group work.

All sessions are evaluated by the participants and the peer educators through a brief questionnaire.

Dorset

DORSET SUBSTANCE MISUSE PREVENTION GROUP

Park Lodge, Gloucester Road, Boscombe, Dorset BH7 6JF

Tel: 01202 397003   **Fax:** 01202 399649

Contact: Tony Deavin

Main business: Advice, support, information

EDDAS (EAST DORSET DRUG AND ALCOHOL SERVICE)

28 Poole Hill, Bournemouth, Dorset BH2 5PS

Tel: 01202 311606   **Fax:** 01202 311777

Contact: Margaret Cunningham

Health authority: Dorset

Other drug services: Training; advice, counselling and befriending organisation

Drug and Alcohol Awareness

This initiative aims: to provide education on drugs and alcohol, dispelling myths and fallacies; to highlight the risks and dangers involved; and to promote the advice and support agency.

Contact: Margaret Cunningham

Tel: 01202 311606

Funders: Health Authority, Social Services

Target age groups: 11 and over

Target group: Parents

Methods: Education is offered through the use of videos, discussion, questionnaires, games, brainstorming, leaflets, and posters.

SOUTH WESSEX ADDICTION SERVICE

202 Holdenhurst Road, Bournemouth, Dorset BH8 8AS

Tel: 01202 552266   **Fax:** 01202 315516

Contact: Mary Cummings

Health authority: Dorset

Other drug services: Treatment; criminal justice; training; counselling; therapy groups; aftercare; schools work and other educative activities

Drug and Alcohol Awareness

This initiative aims: to explore attitudes to drugs; to raise self-esteem around the misuse of substances; to provide education on drugs; to develop refusal skills; and to promote healthy lifestyles.

Contact: Mary Cummings

Tel: 01305 552266

Partner: Mobile health team (occasionally)

Funders: Health/Social Services; charitable donations

Target age groups: 11 and over

Target groups: Not at school; children in care; parents

Methods: Brainstorming, discussion, questionnaires, small group work, and peer support are all offered.

DDAS (DORSET DRUGS AND ALCOHOL ADVISORY SERVICE)

83 The Esplanade, Weymouth, Dorset DT4 7AA

Tel: 01305 760799   **Fax:** 01305 789030

Contact: Chris Snelling

Health authority: Dorset

Other drug services: Treatment; criminal justice; training; community care and support

Drug awareness sessions

The aim of the sessions is: to provide factual information regarding drugs and to highlight the risks and dangers involved; and to look at attitudes to drugs, and how to resist the social pressures to take them.

Contact: Chris Snelling

Tel: 01305 760799

Funders: Health Authority; Social Services

Target age groups: 11–18

Target group: Those with learning difficulties

Methods: The services educate through brainstorming, questionnaires, and discussion groups.

Gloucestershire

GLOUCESTERSHIRE CONSTABULARY

Police HQ, Lansdown Road, Cheltenham, Gloucestershire GL51 6HQ

Tel: 01242 276328   **Fax:** 01242 2221415

Contact: Chief Inspector David Reid

Health authority: Gloucestershire

Other drug services: Treatment; community safety; criminal justice; inter-agency referral

Main business: Drug work as an important aspect of much wider policing activities

Drugs awareness education

This education is delivered mainly, but not exclusively, in schools. It is based on providing information on drug and substance issues to young people to enable them to make informed decisions.

Contact: Police Constable Steve Grimsley

Tel: 01242 524848

Partners: Local Education Authority; schools

Funders: Gloucestershire Constabulary; Gloucestershire Local Education Authority; Drug Education and Prevention

Target age groups: 11–16

Target groups: Parents (Parent–Teacher Associations); neighbourhoods

Methods and evaluation: The work of the project is educating and providing information.

Evaluation was commissioned from another department in the Gloucestershire Constabulary and took the form of participant questionnaires, of which almost 100 were completed.

YOUNG GLOUCESTERSHIRE – THE INFOBUZZ

Peter Scott House, 78 London Road, Gloucester GL1 3PG

Tel: 01452 520048   **Fax:** 01452 380243

Contact: Michelle Stephens

Health authority: Gloucestershire

Main business: Providing personal development, training and leisure opportunitites for young people, and supporting the organisations and groups to which they belong

The Infobuzz Mobile Information Project

This is a mobile information project for young people aged 11–25 in Gloucestershire, which provides information relating to drugs, alcohol and sexual health. It aims to provide young people with a range of information to enable them to make informed choices about their lifestyles; access to trained workers; and signposting to other agencies/organisations.

Contact: Michelle Stephens

Tel: 01452 520048

Partners: Alcohol Counselling and Information Service; Gloucestershire Constabulary; Gloucestershire Crime Prevention Unit/Panel; Gloucestershire Drug Education and Prevention; Gloucestershire Health Promotion Unit/Service

Funders: Variety of charitable trusts

Target age groups: 11–25

Target group: Neighbourhoods

Methods and evaluation: The project is based in a converted coach, housing information displays, leaflets and video presenters. A computer database is currently being established. It is staffed by a group of experienced workers from a variety of professional backgrounds, including nursing, social work and youth work. The Buzz visits venues, and young people are free to access the Buzz to collect leaflets, watch a video or talk with staff. If young people request further help, they are directed to appropriate agencies. At youth clubs there are discussion groups, quizzes, etc.

Ongoing evaluation involves counting the numbers who use the project. Questionnaires are sent to young people using the project and to people making the bookings. Worker evaluation sheets are completed at the end of a session.

THE CLOCKTOWER PROJECT

Tower Road North, Warmley, Gloucestershire BS15 2XU

Tel: 0117 967 1655

Contact: Gillian Anderson

Health authority: Avon

Main business: Youth and community work with girls and women

Drop-in project

The aim of this project is: to provide a safe, confidential service; to offer accessible information/advice; to encourage critical reflection of drugs use; and to equip young women with drugs prevention skills.

Contact: Gillian Anderson

Tel: 0117 967 1655

Funders: Crime Prevention

Needs assessment methods: A survey was carried out in 1992. Also, feedback from a drug action project revealed hidden drug use among young women, particularly young mothers.

Target age groups: 17 and over

Target group: Neighbourhoods

Methods: The project provides a drop-in centre to enable young women to access information, advice and support. Activities are offered (e.g. photography) if needed. This is a brand new project, so will run according to expressed needs.

Young Women's Drug Project

The project aims to raise girls' drugs awareness and has created a leaflet written by young women for young women. It is also working on creating posters to look at positive ways to say no to drugs.

Contact: Tina Bond

Tel: 0117 967 1655

Funders: Bristol Drug Prevention Team; Clocktower Association

Target age groups: 11–21

Methods and evaluation: The project visits other youth centres, with the main base being Clocktower, and uses a whole range of leaflets and information to educate and inform. Participants wrote a booklet (1000 printed) and card inserts. Now looking at positive images of young women and drugs – how to say no – for posters, which will be offered for sale. It also uses current information, discussion groups, photography, peer education and multi-media.

The first part of the project (booklet only) was evaluated for the funders. A worker interviewed girls, participants, and professionals in the area.

Hampshire

DOTS (DRUGS ON THE STREETS) PEER TRAINING PROJECT

5 Pickford Street, Aldershot, Hampshire GU11 1TY

Tel: 01252 311786   **Fax:** 01252 310374

Contact: Lesley Buckland

Health authority: North and Mid Hampshire

DOTS video and teaching pack

The video was produced entirely by young people, so aims to have more credibility with the audience, which is young people aged 11–16 years. A working party consisting of: health specialists a personal health and social education co-ordinator, teachers, a peer training co-ordinator and peer trainers worked on the teaching pack, aimed at Key Stages 3 and 4 in the drug guidelines of the national curriculum.

Contact: Lesley Buckland

Tel: 01252 311786

Partners: Hampshire Youth Service; Rushmoor and Hart Borough Council; Hampshire Constabulary; Health Promotion Unit/Service; Acorn Community Drug Advisory Service; youth clubs of Hampshire and the Isle of Wight

Funders: The Bishop of Guildford's Foundation; Hart Borough Council

Needs assessment methods: One of the objectives of the Drug Action Team area is to get better drugs resources into schools, as there are not many good drugs resources that have credibility with young people.

Target age groups: 11–16

Methods: As a way to access schools and youth projects further afield sponsorship was obtained to make a video of one of the plays in the roadshow. The video also includes interviews with young people who: have never used illegal drugs; have used drugs but have now stopped; or have friends who have used drugs. The peer trainers were trained to use the video equipment and were involved in every stage of producing the video. A teaching pack accompanies the video.

Drug Awareness Roadshow

The roadshow aims to raise awareness of the dangers of substance misuse by providing accurate information and thus enabling young people to make informed choices. The roadshow consists of: a piece of theatre carrying harm prevention messages, workshops/discussions on substance misuse; T-shirts carrying harm minimisation messages.

Contact: Lesley Buckland

Tel: 01252 311786

Funders: North and Mid Hampshire Health Commission; Hampshire Crime Prevention Unit/Panel, Rushmoor Borough Council

Needs assessment methods: Survey on substance misuse among young people in the area.

Target age groups: 11–21

Target groups: Not at school; rural communities

Methods and evaluation: Five linked training days and two residentials are held, including sessions on: research; team building; learning styles/skills; communication techniques; and role-play.

Monitoring forms are completed by: peer trainers, young people, youth workers, and staff.

BASINGSTOKE COMMUNITY DRUG SERVICE

Speciality Services, 8 Fairfields Road, Basingstoke, Hampshire RG25 3DR

Tel: 01256 469006   **Fax:** 01256 331469

Contact: Sarah Baines

Health authority: North and Mid Hampshire

Other drug services: Treatment; training; outreach, research and development

Drug prevention and information service

The service aims to inform, educate and hopefully prevent the uptake of drugs by young people; it also informs parents of what to look for and how to deal with situations.

Contact: Graeme Nice

Tel: 01256 469006

Funders: Loddon NHS Trust

Target age groups: 11 and over

Target groups: Homeless; parents; neighbourhoods; rural communities

Methods and evaluation: A peer education project was carried out in three colleges with parent drugs awareness evenings. Other activities include: work with young people, visit/talks to youth clubs, schools, groups; drugs information bus visits to schools, etc.

Evaluation is through an anonymous questionnaire.

SW FOREST PEER-LED EDUCATION PROJECT

Youth Centre – New Milton, Culver Road, New Milton, Hampshire BH25 6SY

Tel: 01425 616694   **Fax:** 01425 628530

Contact: Jane Finan

Health authority: Southampton and South West Hampshire

Main business: To promote equality of opportunity and offer educational, participative, and empowering opportunities in informal settings for young people in the 11–25 age range

SW Forest Peer-Led Project

The project involves peer-led education with 14–21-year-olds in youth settings, and raises issues of alcohol and substance abuse affecting young people's lives at home, work, and during leisure time, in order to provide them with greater knowledge and enable them to make informed choices.

Contact: Jane Finan

Tel: 01425 616694

Funders: South West Hampshire and Southampton Health Commission; Hampshire County Youth Service

Needs assessment methods: Consultations with youth groups and individual young people in the area through questionnaires, discussion and workshops.

Target age groups: 11 and over

Target groups: Offenders; neighbourhoods; rural communities

Methods and evaluation: Core peer educators were recruited, and consultation and negotiation of a training programme followed. This took the form of workshops, events, planning, preparation, and evaluation with young people and project workers. Training sessions were based on information gained from local young people. After delivery, evaluation and a celebration took place. The core group are now planning recruitment for year 2.

The core group of peer educators evaluated their individual work by producing files containing evidence of their work. Main events were evaluated in written form against aims and objectives set, as well as through discussion and noted/observed learning outcomes. The project was evaluated in January and again at the end of March 1996, against the original aims and objectives.

COMMITMENT TO YOUTH

Community Relations, Police Headquarters, West Hill, Winchester, Hampshire SO22 5DB

Tel: 01962 868133   **Fax:** 01962 843113

Contact: Inspector Ray Hulks

Health authority: North and Mid Hampshire

Other drug services: Community safety; criminal justice; training; referral to support agencies

Main business: Promoting community safety through community partnerships.

Global Rock Challenge

The Global Rock Challenge is an entertainment and youth cultural event: a friendly performing arts competition between secondary schools and youth groups, providing young people with an opportunity to produce and stage a piece of live entertainment.

Contact: Chief Inspector Mark Pontin

Tel: 01962 868133

Partner: Hampshire and Isle of Wight Local Education Authority

Funders: Portsmouth Safer Cities; Radio Victor, Hampshire County Council

Target age groups: 11 and over

Target group: Offenders

Methods: The Rock Challenge encourages teenagers around the world to live a healthy lifestyle. It aims: to deliver substance abuse prevention messages and activites; to teach in a positive way that excellence is achieved through application of creativity, hard work, enthusiasm and co-operation; and to assist in the education process by increasing self-esteem through a positive, fun experience.

Hertfordshire

DRUGLINK LTD

Trefoil House, Red Lion Lane, Hemel Hempstead, Hertfordshire HP3 9TE

Tel: 01923 260727   **Fax:** 01923 260733

Contact: Sandy Durham

Health authority: West Hertfordshire

Other drug services: Treatment; criminal justice

Peer education on safer dancing

The project aims to train 16–18-year-olds in drugs information, health issues and emergency action, with the aim of their passing on the information and advice to peers.

Contact: Greg Green

Tel: 01923 260733

Partner: Urban Access (youth counselling)

Funders: Youth and community service, Hertfordshire; local nightclubs

Target age groups: 11 and over

Target groups: Users of heroin, amphetamines, dance drugs

Methods and evaluation: The project uses crisis counselling and first aid. Ten peer educators were trained during a six-week course and they then passed on the information to their friends and family. They were also taken to nightclubs and other events to look after the welfare of recreational drug users. As support the peer educators receive regular supervision from trained drug workers.

Interviews and questionnaires were used to evaluate the training given to the volunteers, and to see what level of support they required in the long term.

COMMUNITY DRUG AND ALCOHOL TEAM (WATFORD)

18 Upton Road, Watford, Hertfordshire WD1 7EP

Tel: 01923 255124   **Fax:** 01923 241120

Contact: Andy Bishop

Health authority: Hertfordshire

Other drug services: Treatment; criminal justice; training

Court outreach

Outreach is provided for young people who are involved in the criminal justice system and drug use, and who are attending juvenile court.

Contact: Allison Squirrell

Tel: 01923 255124

Partners: Young persons' team; probation team

Target groups: Offenders; minority ethnic groups; not at school; homeless; children in care; parents; neighbourhoods; those at risk of custodial sentence

Methods: Assessment is a condition of treatment. Leaflets are provided, putting young people in touch with other services – youth counselling, careers or counselling assessment. Also work in supporting social workers, and in assessment for rehabilitation.

HERTFORDSHIRE DRUG EDUCATION FORUM

The Education Centre, Butterfield Road, Wheathampstead, Hertfordshire AL4 8PY

Tel: 01582 830341   **Fax:** 01582 830290

Contact: Pauline Barker

Health authority: Hertfordshire

Isle of Wight

IoW DRUG PREVENTION IN SCHOOLS PROJECT

Health Education Unit, 126 Pyle Street, Newport, Isle of Wight PO30 1JW

Tel: 01983 528817   **Fax:** 01983 826099

Contact: Janice Slough

Health authority: Isle of Wight

Other drug services: Training

IoW Parent Week

This project aims to inform and support parents whilst helping them to develop further parenting skills. It offers workshops, in-depth parent support groups and one-to-one work.

Contact: Helen Blake

Tel: 01983 528817

Funder: Local Education Authority

Needs assessment methods: Meetings were held with all agencies working with parents and questionnaires were completed by parents and professionals.

Target groups: Parents; neighbourhoods

Methods and evaluation: One-to-one support and help, usually in a crisis as well as workshops in schools and the community and support groups in the community.

The project is being evaluated and funded by Grants for Education Support and Training (GEST).

Evaluation by GEST and the independent evaluator is continuous.

Kent

YOUTH ACTION 2000

Support Office, Phoenix Youth Centre, Hawes Lane, West Wickham, Kent BR4 9AE

Tel: 0181 777 7938   **Fax:** 0181 777 1914

Contact: Gwendoline Jones

Health authority: Bromley

Other drug services: Community safety; criminal justice; training

Main business: A youth provision to young people in the north-west area of Bromley

Diversion activities

These activities involved informal and social education around the misuse of crack. They aim to educate young people, as well as youth workers, in preparation for a peer-education project.

Contact: Julie Hayward

Tel: 0181 676 8805

Partners: Youth Awareness Programme; Lewisham Drugs Line

Funders: Bromley Drugs Health Authority; Youth Action 2000; Crystal Palace

Needs assessment methods: A report on the change in young people's moods revealed young people asking for support.

Target age groups: 11–21

Target groups: Black Caribbean; black African; users of crack/cocaine; community groups (near housing estates); young people living in isolation

Methods and evaluation: The project provides funding for people who live independently and challenges young men about the misuse of drugs, using sport to increase their awareness of the effects that drugs have on their bodies. A peer-education programme will take place with staff and young people when funding is found.

Evaluation is through the assessment of whether young people are participating in the sports activity, and are being diverted and supported away from drug misuse.

Drop-in for local young people

This initiative involved discussing unemployment and drug use with local young people, and raising young people's awareness about the long- and short-term effects of drugs. The activities ran until January 1996

Contact: Lisa Mayhead

Tel: 0181 658 9663

Partner: Bromley Advisory Information Service (BAIS)

Funders: Youth Action 2000; BAIS

Needs assessment methods: The needs of young people were assessed during informal contact time by youth workers.

Target age groups: 11–21

Target group: Neighbourhoods

Methods and evaluation: The initiative used a video to start discussions, and continued with handing out information about particular drugs, information on the law and drug use, and information on dance drugs, in particular how to help a friend in need. There was a discussion on myths of drug effects, and quizzes and word searches.

Evaluation was carried out by staff and directors of Youth Action 2000, by a youth worker and a BAIS outreach worker, who looked at the aims and objectives of the project.

Peer-Led Young People Drug Awareness Project

The project aims to educate a group of young people around the issue of illegal drug use. The group includes those who do and do not take or use illegal drugs, and is also mixed in terms of culture, gender, class and ability. The programme involves six meetings (residential, three days) and an evaluation meeting.

Contact: Gwen Jones

Tel: 0181 777 7938

Partners: Bromley Health Authority; DrugLink – Lewisham

Funder: Bromley Health Authority

Target age groups: 11–21

Target groups: Offenders; black African; not at school; homeless; children in care; neighbourhoods; community groups

Methods: Currently young people have met three times with youth workers, who facilitate ice-breaking games. Discussions of personal details take place, in confidence, about drug taking. One young person has chosen not to take illegal drugs at all. All meetings are recorded and typed up for everyone. A programme and venue for residential, young person-led, fun activities, e.g. horseriding, canoeing, and workshops with drug awareness trainer were discussed. Young people are looking at resources, literature, books and videos to take to the New Forest. Guidelines, e.g. confidentiality, rules around illegal/legal drugs at the weekend, and respect for personal views were also worked on.

Lancashire

SOLVENT ABUSE RESOURCE GROUP

28 Penny Street, Blackburn, Lancashire BB1 6HL

Tel: 01254 677493 **e-mail:** sarg@airtime.co.uk

Contact: Keith Owen

Health authority: East Lancashire

Other drug services: Treatment; community safety; criminal justice; training; community development

Solvent Abuse Resource Group

This group provides free and confidential help, information and guidance to users, parents, friends and anyone who is interested or concerned about the issue of solvent and/or other substance misuse by young people.

Contact: Keith Owen

Tel: 01254 677493

Funders: National Lottery Charities Board; Blackburn Council; East Lancashire Health Authority, Department of Health, Lancashire County Council

Target group: Users of solvents

BYPASS (BOLTON YOUNG PEOPLE'S ADVICE AND SUPPORT SERVICE)

106–108 Newport Street, Bolton, Lancashire BL3 6AB

Tel: 01204 362002   **Fax:** 01204 388982

Contacts: Peter Little, Marilyn Davies

Health authority: Wigan and Bolton

Main business: Drop-in and advice centre; confidential counselling; sexual health; housing; advocacy

BYPASS Drug Support Project

This is an induction and training programme that equips young people with the necessary skill to provide (in a voluntary capacity) peer group support to those who need help and advice around drug issues.

Contact: Marilyn Davies

Tel: 01204 362002

Funders: Save the Children Fund; Home Office Drug Prevention Initiative

Needs assessment methods: These were carried out during the project.

Methods: The project worker: designs a training programme for young people to provide peer group support; delivers a training programme to volunteers at BYPASS; provides ongoing support to volunteers; develops an advice and information system around drug issues; delivers sessional advice and support to BYPASS users; reviews available training materials; carries out consultation with young people to find out what training and support they require; and reviews and accesses available drug information.

CLITHEROE DRUG PREVENTION PARTNERSHIP

Trinity Centre, Wesleyan Row, Parson Lane, Clitheroe, Lancashire BB7 2JY

Tel: 01200 427886   **Fax:** 01200 285543

Contact: Christopher May

Health authority: East Lancashire

Other drug services: Training; support for parents of drug users; networking

Education and support work with parents

The aim of the work is to develop a support group for parents of drug users and to provide participant education sessions for parents who are concerned about drugs.

Contact: Chris May

Tel: 01200 427886

Partners: Lancashire County Council; youth and community service

Funders: East Lancashire Health authority; Lancashire County Council

Target groups: Parents; community groups

Methods and evaluation: Parents are involved in a support group by the efforts of community-based networking/outreach/publicity. The work delivers sessions on raising awareness and action planning to existing community groups. There is a 24-hour advice and information line (answerphone).

An evaluation sheet is completed by parents in contact with support service. Evaluations are also completed by participants in education sessions, and staff evaluate the objectives for each session.

Targeted work with young people

The work involves providing education, advice and support to young people who are thought to be using drugs, with a view to reducing the harm associated with drug use.

Contact: Chris May

Tel: 01200 427886

Partner: Lancashire Youth and Community Service

Funders: East Lancashire Health Authority; Lancashire County Council

Target group: Drug users

Methods and evaluation: Contact is made with young people in youth clubs or on outreach in local parks. One-to-one interventions, support and information follows through daytime sessions involving discussion and art-based activity. There is a residential weekend offering information development and peer education through information design.

Evaluation is through group discussion, personal interview and questionnaire.

HEALTH PROMOTION SERVICE

Ormskirk Hospital, Wigan Road, Ormskirk, Lancashire L39 2AZ

Tel: 01695 583019   **Fax:** 01695 583018

Contact: Jackie Griffin-Lea

Health authority: South Lancashire

Other drug services: Treatment; community safety; training; health promotion; community development

Main business: Health care and promotion

Skelmersdale Drug Forum

This is a multi-agency forum focusing on parent education and empowerment, and presently developing a theatre and video project. Its aim is to reduce harm associated with drug misuse.

Contact: Jackie Griffin-Lea

Tel: 01695 583019

Partners: Residents associations; voluntary sector; NHS trust; Health Promotion Unit/ Service; police; probation service; District Council, youth service; colleges

Target groups: Neighbourhoods; Skelmersdale community groups; rural communities

Methods and evaluation: A theatre project is being developed to take interactive and empowering drugs/alcohol awareness to parents. It is also to be translated on to video and made available to local parents.

The performance has been previewed and feedback gathered from the audience.

DRUGLINE – LANCASHIRE

2 Union Court, Union Street, Preston, Lancashire PR1 2HD

Tel: 01772 253840   **Fax:** 01772 887927

Contact: Kathryn Talboys

Health authority: North West Lancashire

Other drug services: Treatment; training

Dance Drug Safety

Personnel are available at local dance venues with information, support and appropriate literature.

Contact: Kathryn Talboys

Tel: 01772 253840

Partners: Preston Community Drug Team; North West Lancashire Health Promotion Unit/Service; Community Outreach Project

Funders: Community Health Fund; North West Lancashire Health Promotion Unit/Service; World AIDS Day

Needs assessment methods: Carried out at gay venues in Blackpool and Preston revealing drug use, lack of available appropriate information, and fear of agencies.

Target group: Users of dance drugs; gay community

Methods and evaluation: Generic dance drug safety is undertaken at local clubs, with workers and appropriate information available, as well as a noted presence through an unstaffed stall. A liaison is also undertaken with club owners to encourage safety, and with security/bouncers regarding practical safety.

Evaluation is on gay men's work only, through questionnaires completed by community members, forum members, events volunteers and oral feedback. Generic dance drug safety is evaluated by oral feedback, staff feedback and de-briefing.

Drugs Awareness

This initiative utilises quizzes, exercises, leaflets, games and videos to enhance basic drugs knowledge, improve choices and access to services, improve negotiation skills, and challenge stereotypes of drug use and drug users. Designed to meet the needs of groups, including young people, carers, workers and communities.

Contact: Kathryn Talboys

Tel: 01772 253840

Partners: Local Education Authority; school consortia; university; colleges; community drug team; Health Promotion Unit/Services; community groups

Funders: Joint finance

Target groups: Offenders; black Caribbean; black African; black other; Indian; Pakistani; Bangladeshi; users of dance drugs, anabolic steroids; parents; neighbourhoods; community groups; gay community

Methods and evaluation: Drugline uses a drug training pack which covers facts, attitudes, language and the law. Drugs game is an experiential tool to help understand drug-using lifestyle; Joe Blagg is an experiential tool to build and expand on a drug user/their life/problems faced. The initiative has devised materials to meet specific needs, e.g. for gay/African/Caribbean/Asian communities. It uses presentations, group work, discussions, and bought-in materials, e.g. leaflets, videos and training packs.

Evaluation is through questionnaires, verbal feedback.

NORTH WEST LANCASHIRE HEALTH PROMOTION UNIT

Sharoe Green Hospital, Sharoe Green Lane, Fulwood, Preston, Lancashire PR2 8DU

Tel: 01772 711773   **Fax:** 01772 711113

Contact: Dominic Harrison

Health authority: North West Lancashire

Drugs and Young Sex Workers Project

Project aims to provide early intervention and harm minimisation information to young drug-using sex workers, and to act as advocates into services, while working with services to improve accessibility. The project ran until April 1996.

Contacts: Alayne Robin, Mark Buckley

Tel: 01772 711773

Partners: Community Safety Team/Unit; police; social services; Drugline – Lancashire (see p.116); youth community service

Funders: Young People at Risk from Drugs (DoH grant scheme)

Needs assessment methods: Needs identified with sex workers using 'snowballing' contact methods to identify health needs, with specific focus on sexual health. Review of related research in neighbouring localities.

Target age groups: 11 and over

Target groups: Homeless; neighbourhoods

Methods and evaluation: The project provided mediation and advocacy information services, as well as street level provision of resources for harm minimisation. A community development model was used with detached outreach work to contact the initial target group – drug-using sex workers. Contact was made through 'snowballing' methods, assisted by ex-users on the outreach team. The target location was systematically identified in the second half of the project, together with the dissemination of promotion materials specific to the project through appropriate access points. The contact 'circle' was broadened to include drug-using young people who were possibly vulnerable to becoming involved in sex work. The target groups were young women and men in liaison with the outreach project.

Evaluation was carried out by an independent evaluator for Young People at Risk from Drugs, and there was also an evaluation report by the project team.

Evaluation took the form of process and outcome. The key outcomes reflected models used, and strategies were developed for delivering a short term project with a 'hard to access' group. Furthermore, strategies were developed for contacting and monitoring activity, and for the development of a health carer model for early intervention with the target group.

THE EARLY BREAK DRUGS PROJECT

Ash Tree Barn, Coal Pit Lane, Waterfoot, Rossendale, Lancashire BB4 9SA

Tel: 01706 229537   **Fax:** 01706 226992

Contact: Ian Clements

Health authority: Bury and Rochdale

Other drug services: Treatment; training; support for parents

Early intervention work with young users

Activities centre on providing a drugs service to under-18s and parents, as well as running peer education work.

Contact: Ian Clements

Tel: 01706 229537

Partners: Bury Health Authority; Bury Local Education Authority

Funders: Early Break; Health Authority; Grants for Education Support and Training (GEST)

Target age groups: 11–18

Target groups: Not at school; children in care; parents

Methods and evaluation: Early Break works face-to-face with young people who use drugs, offering them support, counselling, referral information, etc. The peer education work is a partnership project with the police, the Health Authority, and the Local Education Authority to work in high schools and to develop student assisted programmes. Grants for Education Support and Training (GEST) support innovative projects.

Evaluation is through interviews with past and present service users. There is also a forum for training courses.

Leicestershire

LEICESTERSHIRE CRIMEBEAT

Leicestershire Crimebeat, PO Box 482, Leicester LE99 1AY

Tel: 0116 248 2482   **Fax:** 0116 248 2537

Contact: Vivienne Brenchley

Health authority: Leicestershire

Other drug services: Community safety; crime prevention

Main business: Empowerment of young people

Crownhills Senior Club

The aim of the club was to continue learning about drugs and the issues surrounding them. The project was completed by May 1996.

Contact: Caroline Churchill

Tel: 0116 273 9260

Funders: Department for Education and Employment; Crimebeat

Target groups: Offenders; neighbourhoods

Methods: Members took part in a weekend away with a theme of drug awareness, building on past workshops. Participants had the idea of making a video looking at the issues raised to show at other youth centres. Advisers/trainers from the local drug action team attended to discuss facts and look at risk management. Follow-up work continued at college.

More Than A Feeling

This is a video based on the format of a role-playing adventure book (14 storylines possible), in which viewers learn about drugs, alcohol, solvents, etc.

Contact: Nigel Roberts

Tel: 01530 560940

Partners: East Midlands Drug Fund; Police Partnership

Funders: Ashby Educational Fund; East Midlands Drug Fund, Crimebeat, East Midlands Arts

Target groups: Offenders; parents of school goers

Methods: Viewers are able to watch different story lines and decide on a course of action. Once a choice is made, the viewer can fast forward to the next scene to see the consequences of their decision. Advice is provided on screen by experts from doctors to the police. The production was devised, designed, made and produced by young people under 25 years.

LEICESTERSHIRE DRUG ADVICE CENTRE

Paget House, 2 West Street, Leicester LE1 6XP

Tel: 0116 247 0200   **Fax:** 0116 247 1600

Contact: Trevor McCarthy

Health authority: Leicestershire

Other drug services: Treatment; community safety; criminal justice; training

Asian and African-Caribbean Peer EDP

Aims to further links and networking with Asian and African-Caribbean communities in Leicestershire; to build up a group/network of young Asian and African-Caribbean people who are able to educate and pass on their knowledge to others; to contribute through documentation and evaluation to further relevant education and prevention work with Asian and African-Caribbean young people.

Contacts: Deborah Sangster, Kirit Mistry

Tel: 0116 247 0200

Partners: East Midlands Drug Prevention Team

Funders: Leicestershire Social Services: Leicestershire Health Authority

Needs assessment methods: The Leicestershire Drug Advice Centre's African-Caribbean project worker and Asian project worker made direct contact with young black people in a range of settings – including schools, estates and projects. This highlighted the need for educational approaches tailored to the needs and context of black people. The workers also consulted with black workers in a range of educational/ welfare settings, and identified that there needed to be a fresh and personalised approach to developing work with black communities.

Target age groups: 11 and over

Target groups: Black Caribbean; black African; black other; Indian; Pakistani; Bangladeshi

Methods and evaluation: The training programme for the peer educators consists of 10 three-hour weekly sessions plus a residential weekend course. The course was organised around four core elements: personal development; street drug awareness; facilitation skills; and society, drugs and black communities. Following completion of the course, participants, on a voluntary basis, undertake drug educational activities on a formal or informal basis with other black (and white) young people.

The project is being externally evaluated by an independent researcher appointed by the East Midlands Drug Prevention Initiative. The training programme for the peer educators was accredited by the Open College Network.

There are also post programme interviews.

Safe and Sound – drugs education project

The project aims to: improve the access of young people to both information and opportunities; consider the implications of drug use through working with youth workers; and provide direct education about drugs and risks.

Contact: Bo Deyall

Tel: 0116 247 0200

Partners: Leicestershire Local Education Authority; youth and community section

Funders: Leicestershire Drug Advice Centre; Leicestershire Local Education Authority

Needs assessment methods: Prior to the project as a whole, there was discussion with young people and youth workers which indicated the low input of active, focused drugs education.

Target age groups: 11 and over

Methods and evaluation: Two part-time sessional workers (supervised by a full-time development worker) on the staff of Leicestershire Drug Advice Centre work with young people's projects on a twice weekly basis for a month. Methods used in sessions with young people include: mini-inputs on drugs/issues, writing songs/poetry, video, art/collage, quizzes, debates; and role-plays.

Evaluation is informal and by participants and staff. It includes quizzes, value change/choice activities, 'walls' on which young people can write or draw, conversations with young people and youth workers, and workers' recordings of planning, running and reviewing sessions.

SAFFRON YOUNG PEOPLE'S PROJECT (SYPP)

432 Saffron Lane, Leicester LE2 6SB

Tel: 0116 283 1765

Contact: Jay Stewart

Health authority: Leicestershire

Main business: Detached youth work; action research

Detached youth work/action research

SYPP aims to work with young people rather than upon them. Within this, SYPP aims to challenge misinformation and the social taboo surrounding drug use, and to stimulate open and informed debate among young people and the wider community.

Contact: Jay Stewart

Tel: 0116 283 1765

Funders: Drug Prevention Initiative; city and county council, Saffron Neighbourhood Council

Needs assessment methods: An 18-month action research project found that there was a need among young people for a detached youth work project based on a social action approach.

Target age groups: 11 and over

Methods: SYPP responds to young people's needs by discussing with the young the multitude of issues that impact on their lives. In terms of looking at the theme of drug use, young people's involvement in peer education as well as the more general issues of young people's participation and exclusion from society have been the key issues addressed by the project using methods including drama and video.

SPEAKEASY THEATRE COMPANY

30 Upper Tichborne Street, Leicester LE2 1GJ

Tel: 0116 254 4623

Contact: Andy Reeves

Health authority: Leicestershire

Respect 96

This is a drug awareness play for young people, aged 11–13 which provides, through the medium of drama, an entertaining but thought-provoking live experience aimed at promoting health education and safer lifestyle choices in the area of drug use.

Contact: Andy Reeves

Tel: 0116 254 4623

Partners: Leicestershire Constabulary; Local Education Authority; Leicester City Challenge Project; Leicestershire Drug Advice Centre

Funders: Leicester City Challenge Project; Leicestershire Constabulary

Target age groups: 11–13

Methods and evaluation: The play itself contains questions, information and answers about drug use by young people, but in a light-hearted and unthreatening way. Themes developed are: health; social attitudes to legal and illegal drugs; informed choice; and personal safety. These are continued in participatory workshop sessions, where young people interact with the actors through role-playing and putting themselves in imagined scenarios, e.g. 'What would you have done then?', 'Why?', 'What if…?'.

Evaluation took place through written responses from the first audience to see the play.

Lincolnshire

LINCOLNSHIRE HEALTH PROMOTION

Annex C, Council Offices, Eastgate, Sleaford, Lincolnshire NG34 7DP

Tel: 01529 306011   **Fax:** 01529 306121

Contact: Craig Kershaw

Health authority: Lincolnshire

Other drug services: Community safety; training; providing resources

Bus tour

Tying in with the launch of a substance misuse strategy in May (1996), the aim of the bus tour was to raise awareness and disseminate information about the strategy to the people of Lincolnshire from March to May 1996.

Contact: Emma Warr

Tel: 01529 306011

Funders: Community Council; Lincolnshire County Council; Grantham Drugs Awareness; Lincolnshire HIV/AIDS Voluntary Group; Lincolnshire Health Authority

Funders: Lincolnshire Health Authority; Lincolnshire County Council, Grantham Drug Awareness, Lincolnshire Health Authority

Target groups: Rural communities

Methods: Lincolnshire Health Promotion's bus was used to provide the general public and professionals with information about the Lincolnshire substance misuse strategy. The bus toured around the county, and was placed in key locations.

Lincolnshire Drug Prevention Week

The week, with the theme 'Have a safe night', aims to raise awareness of the issues concerning the use/misuse of substances, harm minimisation, issues of peer pressure, and safer behaviour in a variety of settings with young people.

Contact: Jacki Olive

Tel: 01529 306011

Partners: Lincolnshire HIV/AIDS Voluntary Group; GUM clinic; Pilgrim; Grantham youth service

Funders: Lincolnshire Health Promotion; Lincolnshire HIV/AIDS Voluntary Group

Target age groups: 11 and over

Target groups: Neighbourhoods; rural communities

Methods: The Drug Prevention Week includes static and/or mobile displays of drug education material in the form of posters, pamphlets, videos, test-your-knowledge boxes, competitions, quizzes, and group and individual discussion. Activities are directed/facilitated by the outreach team in five town/village centre sites and five nightclub settings countrywide.

Peer education project

This project aims to develop a peer-led education project for young people around drugs and sexual health issues.

Contact: Terry Miller

Tel: 01529 306011

Funders: Lincolnshire Health Authority

Target age groups: 11 and over

Methods: This project is still very much in the planning stage, but it may involve developing a peer education qualification, with awards for differing levels of activity/involvement.

Steroids project

The project involves research into steroid use, the development of resources for bodybuilders/steroid users (including the possible publication of material on harm minimisation/risk reduction, e.g. needle exchange, condom use, and sexual health matters), and an educational strand ('natural' methods of body building).

Contact: Terry Miller

Tel: 01529 306011

Partners: The Health Shop, Lincoln; Association of Natural Bodybuilders

Funders: Lincolnshire Health Authority; Department of Health

Needs assessment methods: Questionnaires have already been developed and distributed, and there may be a focus on group/interview work in the future.

Target group: Users of anabolic steroids

Methods: Information is provided about the side-effects and/or long-term use of anabolic steroids. The project cascades education about safer injecting techniques and safer injecting sites. User-friendly leaflets and posters are distributed to gyms, sport shops, schools, and youth clubs, and there is an involvement of sports organisations devoted to keeping performance-enhancing drugs out of sports.

London

ASIAN DRUG PROJECT (LONDON)

c/o Dame Colet House, Ben Jonson Road, London E1 3NH

Tel: 0171 790 6065

Contact: Shakoth Mial

Health authority: East London and City

Other drug services: Treatment; community safety; training; family and parental support; support in Bengali and Hindi

---

Client advocacy work

This initiative engages, through assessment and referral, members of the drug-using community who seek/need help.

Contact: Mukssod Shaikh

Tel: 0171 790 6065

Funder: Health Authority

Needs assessment methods: Community and professionals were consulted, and 'An Assessment of the Young Bengali Community' was drawn up.

Target groups: Offenders; Indian; Pakistani; Bangladeshi; homeless

Education and counselling for under 17s

The work centres on: awareness of issues around drug use and abuse, referral, advice and one-to-one work; training for youth workers and teachers on Asian approaches to drugs prevention.

Contact: Shakoth Maih

Tel: 0171 790 6065

Funders: Health Authority; social services, Single Regeneration Budget; Crime Prevention

Needs assessment methods: Consultation with young people, clients, families and professionals.

Target groups: Offenders; Indian; Pakistani; Bangladeshi; not at school; homeless; parents

BRIXTON DRUG PROJECT

142 Stockwell Road, London SW9 9TQ

Tel: 0171 502 9819 **e-mail:** allat@brixdrug.demon.co.uk

Health authority: Lambeth, Southwark and Lewisham

Other drug services: Treatment; community safety; criminal justice; training; counselling

Drugs awareness presentations

The presentations give local young people accurate, up-to-date information about illegal drugs and their effects in order to minimise harm to young people using drugs, and to inform young people about relevant drug services and how to access them.

Contact: Arabella Yapp

Tel: 0171 501 9817

Funders: Brixton Challenge; Lambeth Social Services

Needs assessment methods: Schools were given a questionnaire to find out what content they desired in the presentations. The result was that information about drugs, with visual aids to show what they look like, was required.

Target age groups: 11 and over

Target groups: Black Caribbean; black African; black other; not at school; parents; neighbourhoods

Methods: The presentations involve a show of 25 slides covering a wide range of illegal substances and solvents. Each substance and its physical and psychological effects are talked about, and questions are answered. If requested, there are follow-up activities, using a variety of resources and approaches, including a CD-ROM of drug information, music and up-to-date visual effects.

BROMLEY SOMALI COMMUNITY ASSOCIATION

101a Parish Lane, Penge, London SE20 7NR

Tel: 0181 778 5539

Contact: Said Behi Addaid

Health authority: Bromley

Main business: Advice, counselling, representation in immigration, welfare rights and asylum matters

Qat Awareness

The project aims to reduce the consumption and use of Qat by raising awareness among the community of the problems related to it. Leaflets and posters are produced in the Somali language and information sessions on the effects of Qat are held. The project will finish at the end of 1998.

Contact: Said Behi Addaid

Tel: 0181 778 5539

Funder: Supporters

Target groups: Black African; users of Qat, Kaat; not at school; homeless; parents

Methods: People who use Qat are talked to in the streets, parks and community centres about the problems associated with it, and the damage it causes to health as well as financial loss to individuals and the community in general.

CHARTERHOUSE YOUNG PEOPLE CENTRE

40 Tabard Street, London SE1 4JU

Tel: 0171 403 1676   **Fax:** 0171 357 8379

Contact: Julie Bentley

Health authority: Lambeth, Southwark and Lewisham

Other drug services: Training

Main business: Diverse service provision to young people

Drugs/sexual health awareness

This is a peer-education project that aims to provide comprehensive training for young people to increase their skills, knowledge, self-esteem and employment prospects, and to enable them to run drugs and sexual health awareness sessions for their peers.

Contact: Julie Bentley/Simon Claridge

Tel: 0171 403 1676

Partner: Southwark Young People Music Project

Funders: Drug Prevention Team

Target age groups: 11 and over

Target group: Youth workers

Methods and evaluation: The training of the peer-education programme workers and the sessions which they run include: use of group work exercises; role-play; poster design; music and lyrics; pictures of drugs; and games that explore drugs use and effects.

The Policy Studies Institute acts as an external evaluator that interviews staff, participants, and other organisations, and observes actual work.

COMMUNITY SAFETY & PARTNERSHIP BRANCH

Metropolitan Police, New Scotland Yard, Broadway, London SW1H 0BG

Tel: 0171 230 4216   **Fax:** 0171 230 2152

Contact: Inspector Paul Wotton

Health authority: Across London

Other drug services: Community safety; criminal justice; training; referrals to drug agencies

Junior Citizen Scheme

The scheme, known as 'Crucial Crew' outside London, teaches 10–11-year-olds how to cope with everyday dangers safely and effectively by visiting a variety of sites where they are presented with different scenarios, some of which may involve drugs.

Contact: Inspector Bob Jones

Tel: 0171 230 3200

Partners: Police; British Telecom; Gas; Electricity; Fire brigade; Ambulance (St John's); Local authority, e.g. environmental health, parks

Funders: British Telecom; local sponsorship

Needs assessment methods: The scheme addresses local and national needs and complements the Health of the Nation document.

Target groups: Parents; school children

Methods and evaluation: Personal safety is taught. Some schemes identify how to deal with discarded needles, for example.

Each scheme is evaluated locally by staff, and by British Telecom.

Summer Action

This project is aimed at improving relationships, diverting young people away from crime, providing leisure facilities, encouraging partnerships and showing that young people can make a valuable contribution to the community.

Contact: Inspector Bob Jones

Tel: 0171 230 3200

Partners: Midland Bank; police; youth workers; social workers; parents; volunteers; local authority

Funders: Midland Bank; local sponsorship

Needs assessment methods: Summer Action was established in response to local and national needs and is aimed at school summer holiday periods.

Target groups: Offenders; parents (as volunteers); neighbourhoods; community groups (as supporters)

Methods and evaluation: The schemes are based on local estates. Some schemes build in drug prevention overtly while others tackle it more subtly.

Each scheme is evaluated locally by staff and participants, and by the Midland Bank.

Youth Action groups

Groups are held for young people, in which the aim is: to identify a problem that affects them; to identify an activity that may solve it; and to put this activity into action. Some groups have chosen drugs as an issue.

Contact: Inspector Bob Jones

Tel: 0171 230 3200

Partners: Variety of schools and youth services

Funders: Local sponsorship; Crime Concern; Prudential Assurance

Needs assessment methods: The groups were started as a response to local and national needs relating to juvenile offenders, victimisation and active citizenship. It was identified that young people wish to have a voice and to participate.

Target group: Peers

Methods and evaluation: Some groups have completed anonymous questionnaires on the frequency of drug use, while others have conducted prevention campaigns, including the use of drugs. Some have done a survey of the provision (or lack of it) of services for youths in their local area.

The groups are evaluated locally and centrally by staff and participants. Leicester University has evaluated a scheme in Birmingham on behalf of Crime Concern.

EDAS (EALING DRUGS ADVISORY SERVICE)

14 Alexandria Road, London W13 0NR

Tel: 0181 579 1878

Contact: Andi Plastiras

Health authority: Ealing, Hammersmith and Hounslow

Other drug services: Treatment; criminal justice; training; community detoxication service, primary health care; Asian outreach

Youth counselling and information service

The service aimed to contact young people in recreational areas in Ealing in order to promote the service provision in an informal setting offered by the Ealing Youth Counselling and Information Service (EYCIS). The project finished in August 1996.

Contact: Andi Plastiras

Tel: 0181 579 5585

Partners: The Gatehouse Drug Dependency Clinic; Ealing Hospital; EYCIS

Funders: Existing resources

Target age groups: 11 and over

Target groups: Offenders; Indian; Pakistani; Bangladeshi; homeless

Methods: The service aimed to meet with young people in an informal setting, e.g. parks, McDonalds, etc., and to provide access to EYCIS, where information, advice and counselling is available regarding drug use, family, abuse problems, etc.

HIP (HEALTH INFORMATION PROJECT)

336a Ladbroke Grove, London W10 5AS

Tel: 0181 960 5510   **Fax:** 0181 960 6114

Contact: Hugh Dufficy

Health authority: Kensington and Chelsea

Other drug services: Treatment; criminal justice; training

Main business: The project is evenly split between drug work and sexual health work

Drop-in service

This service enables young people and those involved with them to obtain advice and information concerning substance misuse.

Contact: Liz Warrior

Tel: 0181 960 5510

Funders: City Challenge; Kensington and Chelsea youth service

Needs assessment methods: Research was carried out among young people in North Kensington City Challenge area.

Target age groups: 11 and over

Target groups: Offenders; black Caribbean; black African; black other; other minority ethnic groups; not at school; homeless; in care; neighbourhoods

Methods: The drop-in service offers face-to-face advice and information and group discussion among young people using games. The service also distributes appropriate literature.

Educational workshops

Workshops are held for young people on substance use.

Contact: Yvonne Lavine

Tel: 0181 960 5510

Partners: Westminster Drug Project; Riverside Health Outreach Workers; Blenheim Project

Funders: City Challenge; Kensington, Chelsea and Westminster Health Commissioning Agency

Needs assessment methods: Prior to project opening, research was carried out among young people in North Kensington.

Target age groups: 11 and over

Target groups: Offenders; black Caribbean; black African; black other; not at school; homeless; children in care; parents; neighbourhoods; community groups (North Kensington)

Methods and evaluation: Requests are made to the project from organisations requiring workshops. The workshops use participative learning based on the vehicles listed above.

Evaluation is through participants' questionnaires.

Peer education – AfroCaribbean, Moroccan

The aim of this activity is to enable young people to educate others about drug use. The work uses a multi-media approach – music, drama and video art – to develop vehicles that young people can use to discuss drugs and related issues. The activity is to develop one of these areas

Contact: Liz Warrior

Tel: 0181 960 5510

Funders: Kensington, Chelsea and Westminster Health Authority; North Kensington City Challenge; youth services

Needs assessment methods: Research was carried out using questionnaires and one-to-one interviews. Young people in the area wanted an opportunity to learn about drugs in non-formal settings.

Target age groups: 11–21

Target groups: Black Caribbean; black African; black other; neighbourhoods

Methods: Young people are recruited from the street and through drop-in centres. They go through a weekend drug awareness programme: and decide on a vehicle to use and develop material with workers. They are then trained in techniques for how to use the product with other groups. Development of group work and basic training skills are provided, and they are supported by staff to deliver the education.

Peer education – young people

The initiative enables young people to learn about and educate their peers concerning drug use.

Contact: Liz Warrior, Hugh Dufficy

Tel: 0181 960 5510

Funders: City Challenge; Kensington and Chelsea Health Authority

Needs assessment methods: Research questionnaires were completed by, and focus groups held with young people prior to setting up the project.

Target age groups: 11 and over

Methods: The initiative educates a core group of young people about substance use, presentation skills and education. They develop specific learning tools (drama, music, art), chosen by themselves, and present the outcomes at youth clubs and youth-orientated agencies.

Working with Young People: Drug Use

The project runs a basic drug awareness and sexual health awareness course for those working with young people. It also runs a two-day programme which looks in greater detail at managing drug use, and a two-day programme on sexual health within non-specialist settings such as youth clubs, workshops and hostels.

Contact: Hugh Dufficy

Tel: 0181 960 5510

Partners: Kensington and Chelsea youth service; Human Resource Development Unit

Funder: Kensington and Chelsea youth service

Needs assessment methods: Training need analysis was carried out as part of a performance review on the need for basic awareness training and project-specific training on drug use and sexual health.

Target group: Workers with young people

Methods and evaluation: The project works with participative learning, and is evaluated by questionnaires completed by participants.

HOPE UK

25f Copperfield Street, London SE1 0EN

Tel: 0171 928 0848

Contact: Lindsay Taylor

Health authority: Lambeth, Southwark and Lewisham

Alcohol/drug education Bristol and South West

Aims to provide locally available support for primary prevention activities, particularly targeting the voluntary sector and its varied organisations, including parents, and to provide literature and support for the education sector.

Contact: David Wynne

Tel: 0117 961 4454

Partners: Drug reference group; Drug Education and Prevention; Drug Prevention Team

Funders: Hope UK; local trusts and companies; churches; supporters

Target age groups: 11–18

Target group: Parents

Methods and evaluation: Speakers are provided on request to fit in with a group or schools programme. There are several areas offering support: literature – a mixture of free leaflets and a small charge for others; presentations – for parents and other concerned adults; training – for youth workers and church leaders, appropriate to their needs; media – press releases, radio interviews, etc. There are activity-based information/discussion sessions for young people, appropriate to each group's needs as well as exhibitions and displays of work carried out.

The project started as a local pilot in 1990 and formal evaluation took place after 9 and 27 months. Client group opinions were sought and workload measurements used.

Alcohol/drug education East Anglia

The initiative involves the provision of locally available support for primary prevention activities, particularly targeting the voluntary sector and its varied organisations, including parents, and the provision of literature and support for the education sector.

Contact: Andrew Varley

Tel: 01284 753135

Funders: Hope UK; local trusts and companies; churches; supporters

Target age groups: 11–18

Target groups: Parents

Methods and evaluation: Speakers are provided on request to fit in with a group or schools programme. There are several areas offering support: literature – a mixture of free leaflets and a small charge for others; presentations – for parents and other concerned adults; training – for youth workers and church leaders, appropriate to their needs; media – press releases, radio interviews, etc. There are activity-based information/discussion sessions for young people, appropriate to each group's needs as well as exhibitions and displays of work carried out.

Alcohol/drug education Greenwich and Bexley

Aims to provide locally available support for primary prevention activities, particularly targeting the voluntary sector and its varied organisations, including parents, and to provide literature and support for the education sector.

Contact: Hazel Moore

Tel: 0181 317 9240

Partners: Membership of Drug reference group; Health Promotion Unit/Service

Funders: Hope UK; local trusts and companies; churches; supporters

Target age groups: 11–18

Target group: Parents

Methods and evaluation: Speakers are provided on request to fit in with a group or schools programme. There are several areas offering support: literature – a mixture of free leaflets and a small charge for others; presentations – for parents and other concerned adults; training – for youth workers and church leaders, appropriate to their needs; media – press releases, radio interviews, etc. There are activity-based information/discussion sessions for young people, appropriate to each group's needs as well as exhibitions and displays of work carried out.

Alcohol/drug education Plymouth

Aims to provide locally available support for primary prevention activities, particularly targeting the voluntary sector and its varied organisations, including parents, and to provide literature and support for the education sector.

Contact: David Wynne

Tel: 0117 961 4454

Partners: Moorhaven Running Club; Plymouth YMCA

Funders: Hope UK; local trusts and companies; churches; supporters

Target age groups: 11–18

Target group: Parents

Methods and evaluation: Speakers are provided on request to fit in with a group or schools programme. There are several areas offering support: literature – a mixture of free leaflets and a small charge for others; presentations – for parents and other concerned adults; training – for youth workers and church leaders, appropriate to their needs; media – press releases, radio interviews, etc. There are activity-based information/discussion sessions for young people, appropriate to each group's needs as well as exhibitions and displays of work carried out. Annual five-mile run sponsored by Hope UK.

Evaluation takes place through feedback from partner and client groups.

Community-based alcohol/drug education

This is an initiative in Southampton that aims to provide locally available support for primary prevention activities, particularly targeting the voluntary sector and its varied organisations, including parents. It also provides literature and support for the education sector.

Contact: Erika Fullick

Tel: 0170 333 4225

Funders: Hope UK; local trusts and companies; churches

Target age groups: 11–18

Target group: Parents

Methods and evaluation: Speakers are provided on request to fit in with a group or schools programme. There are several areas offering support: literature – a mixture of free leaflets and a small charge for others; presentations – for parents and other concerned adults; training – for youth workers and church leaders, appropriate to their needs; media – press releases, radio interviews, etc. There are activity-based information/discussion sessions for young people, appropriate to each group's needs as well as exhibitions and displays of work carried out.

Getting It Sorted

A series of lessons and activities for 8–12-year-olds, mainly targeting the voluntary sector, provides primary prevention education through games, activities and discussion.

Contact: Tara Russell

Tel: 0171 928 0848

Funders: Hope UK; trusts and companies

Needs assessment methods: During evaluation of existing provision and consultation with teachers and youth workers, the need was identified for such a resource specifically in the voluntary sector, particularly one which also gives leaders' notes.

Target age group: 8–12

Methods: Speakers are provided for schools and youth groups as well as training for leaders in the methods used within the pack. There are opportunities for group discussions about drugs.

Now You Know...

This is a drug education project for 11–14-year-olds that aims to provide effective literature for that age group, and support, advice and resources for those who work with them.

Contact: Christine Hussey

Tel: 0117 961 4454

Partners: British National Temperance League, Sheffield; Amethyst Centre for Alcohol Concern; Lifelink Community Project, Bromley

Funders: Hope UK; DG5 European Union Commission

Needs assessment methods: Interviews with teachers, and youth and church workers in the pilot area (Norfolk).

Target age groups: 11–14

Methods and evaluation: The project provides a booklet, an A1 wallchart, and support packs for teachers, youth workers and church workers.

Evaluation is by questionnaire, mainly completed by participants.

Parents' support project

The project provides information and support for parents and other carers who wish to take steps to encourage their children not to use drugs.

Contact: George Ruston

Tel: 0171 928 0848

Funders: Hope UK; ANSVAR insurance company

Needs assessment methods: Identification of parents as a key target group arose out of Hope UK's planning and review system.

Target group: Parents

Methods and evaluation: The project provides parents with an action plan booklet, and offers presentations to parents in a variety of settings.

There is a short questionnaire for those attending presentations which asks for opinions on the general level of satisfaction and suggestions to help 'fine-tune' the presentations.

Primary drug education for pre-teens

This initiative is based on a series of worksheets and activities aimed at the voluntary sector, mainly church-based groups.

Contact: Tara Russell

Tel: 0171 928 0848

Funders: Hope UK; youth organisations; churches

Target age groups: 8–13

Methods: The initiative uses worksheets, divided into two age groups (8–10s and 11–13s), consisting of practical ideas, games, activities and information. Speakers are provided for groups and churches running a programme. Information leaflets also available.

Volunteer alcohol/drug education

Through this scheme, locally available primary prevention activities are carried out by voluntary workers throughout the UK.

Contact: Sarah Brighton

Tel: 0171 928 0848

Funders: Hope UK

Needs assessment methods: Needs were assessed by identifying target groups for primary prevention; setting objectives for a voluntary worker training scheme; and setting up a monitoring and evaluation system.

Target age groups: 11–21

Target groups: Parents; community groups

Methods and evaluation: Volunteers speak to local groups of all kinds; work with the media; fundraise, mount exhibitions and displays; carry out activity-based information/discussion sessions with young people of all ages; and work with local organisations. They use Hope UK and other literature, and take part in a centrally organised youth roadshow drama event.

Objectives were set as part of the Department for Education and Employment grant agreement for monitoring at set intervals. All those involved took part.

THE HOT ORANGE PROJECT

1a Woolwich New Road, Woolwich, London SE18 6EX

Tel: 0181 855 7673   **Fax:** 0181 854 7689

Contact: Helen Bird

Health authority: Bexley and Greenwich

Other drug services: Treatment

Minimising harm

The project involves interactive training with groups of young people focusing on the risks associated with legal, illegal and illicit drug use. It also offers one-to-one support with alcohol and drug problems, and information and advice at a weekly drop-in.

Contact: Helen Bird

Tel: 0181 855 7673

Funder: Bexley and Greenwich Health Authority

Needs assessment methods: A local survey on the prevalence of substance experimentation was carried out by another organisation, and the need to minimise harm was expressed by young people following after-training evaluation.

Target age group: 11–16

Methods and evaluation: Through outreach work in schools, interactive training methods are used to encourage young people to become aware of the risks involved in substance use. This has enough effect on some young people to discourage them from using drugs. However, harm minimisation messages are also provided which are aimed at those who are or who might experiment in the future. These include continuums, scenarios and brainstorm activities. The project also offers counselling (employing a client-centred approach) with short-term intervention, and a problem-solving approach and a drop-in service (non-judgemental information and advice, and referral to other organisations).

The Hot Orange Project's methods of working in schools was evaluated in 1994–5 by Christchurch College, Canterbury. This was comissioned by the Health Authority.

Training sessions are evaluated through a reflection sheet and the following evaluations also take place: group interviews with students; pre-/post-test quantitative analysis; observation of training sessions; and interviews with staff and teachers.

THE HOXTON TRUST

156 Hoxton Street, London N1 6SH

Tel: 0171 729 1480   **Fax:** 0171 739 6692

Contact: Karina Van Der Merwe

Health authority: East London and City

Main business: Multi-functioning community organisation which began as a development trust 12 years ago and continued to be interested in developing, as well as reflecting, the community needs

Hoxton Trust Outreach Project

The project targets a mixed group of 14–24-year-olds who congregate in and about the Hoxton Trust Community Garden.

Contact: Karina Van Der Merwe

Tel: 0171 729 1480

Partners: Local churches; police; Hackney Local Education Authority

Funders: Department of Health and London Borough of Hackney; Hoxton Trust

Needs assessment methods: Following complaints from parents and local residents who use the garden the Association for the Prevention of Addiction was invited to visit the area, and they reported a need for work to be done. There was evidence of drug use in the garden as well as constant vandalism in the garden and to the trust building.

Target age groups: 11–18

Target groups: Not at school; neighbourhoods

Methods and evaluation: The project has specific targets in terms of the numbers of young people to be contacted; the numbers to show acceptance of the project; the numbers to be individually worked with and the numbers to be returned to education, training or work. Youth workers make contact and then encourage the young people to enter into discussions, play football, and learn a bit more about themselves. Another method is to deal with the group as a whole, and with those who want individual help sometime later.

Evaluation was by a short questionnaire given to 17 people, and a longer one given to a further eight. A report was also produced by an outside agency. Informal discussions are also held.

HUNGERFORD DRUG PROJECT

32a Wardour Street, London W1V 3HJ

Tel: 0171 287 1274

Health authority: Kensington and Chelsea

Other drug services: Training; telephone helpline, drop-in, counselling, shiatsu massage

Detached youth work

This detached work in a variety of locations is targeted at young people who use, have used, or are at risk through the use of illegal drugs.

Contact: Jane Walker

Tel: 0171 287 8743

Partners: Hostels; day centres

Funders: Health Authority; London Borough Grants Unit, London Boroughs of Camden and Islington, Westminster

Target age groups: 17 and over

Target groups: Not at school; homeless; parents; neighbourhoods; young male sex workers

Methods and evaluation: The methods of this project vary according to session and setting, but include: formal education in schools; street and satellite work; and workshops with women's groups and ethnic minority groups.

Evaluation is by the host organisations and participants, and takes the form of self-completed questionnaires; ongoing monitoring; and assessment of intended outcomes.

IMPACT

67–69 Cowcross Street, Farringdon, London EC1M 6BP

Tel: 0171 251 5860   **Fax:** 0171 251 5890

Contact: Janine Rowe

Health authority: Camden and Islington

Other drug services: Treatment; community safety; criminal justice; training

Counselling

This organisation is involved in individual work with young people who are referred to the project. The aim is determined by the service user, with the emphasis on harm minimisation.

Contact: Janine Rowe

Tel: 0171 251 5860

Partners: Schools; health promotions; other organisations

Funders: Various trusts; Local Education Authority

Target age groups: 11–18

Target groups: Offenders; black African; not at school; children in care; parents; neighbourhoods

Methods and evaluation: A referral is arranged with the young person, the referrer (if appropriate), and impact staff. Young persons are offered a comprehensive assessment which includes drug use as well as other relevant areas. Four to six sessions are offered, dependent on the nature of the request and the process is reviewed. Young persons may also be linked with any number of diversionary activities provided by other sources.

Evaluation is by staff, participants and the Department of Health.

THE JUNCTION PROJECT

27 Station Road, London NW10 4UP

Tel: 0181 961 7007   **Fax:** 0181 963 0953

Health authority: Brent and Harrow

Other drug services: Treatment; community safety; criminal justice; training

GP youth worker initiative

The GP youth worker provides advice, information and support to young people on issues such as drugs, alcohol and sexual health.

Contact: Jessica Healy

Tel: 0181 961 7007

Partners: GP surgeries; Brent and Harrow Health Authority

Funders: Young People at Risk from Drugs (DoH grant scheme); Brent and Harrow Health Authority

Target age groups: 11–21

Methods: The GP youth worker takes referrals from GPs in order to provide advice, information and support to young people on issues such as drugs, alcohol and sexual health.

Peer education programme

This programme aims to provide training and ongoing support to groups of young people (15–24 years) who then become a resource to their local communities

Contact: Sandy Campbell

Tel: 0181 961 7007

Funders: Harlesden City Challenge, South Kilburn Single Regeneration Budget

Target age groups: 11 and over

Methods and evaluation: After training, the peer educators are available to their contemporaries for information on a variety of drug-related issues.

The scheme is currently being evaluated by the Centre for Research on Drugs and Health Behaviour.

LEWISHAM INDO-CHINESE COMMUNITY DRUG MISUSE PREVENTION PROJECT

171 High Street, London SE8 3NU

Tel: 0181 692 2772   **Fax:** 0181 691 6815

Contact: V C Truong

Health authority: Lambeth, Southwark and Lewisham

Main business: Community services within Lewisham Indo-Chinese community

Deptford Health Day

The main aim of the project is to educate people about the harmful effects of drugs, and to raise drug awareness in the local community. By participating in activities such as health days, the project can distribute its educational information, and publicise its service.

Contact: Wenxia Ji

Tel: 0181 692 2772

Funders: Various organisations

Needs assessment methods: The future needs of the project are assessed by how many people visit the project stand, how many leaflets are handed out, what age group of people participated, etc.

Target groups: Chinese; other minority ethnic groups; parents; community groups (Indo-Chinese community)

LIFE EDUCATION CENTRE

1st floor, 53–56 Great Sutton Street, London EC1V 0DE

Tel: 0171 490 3210   **Fax:** 0171 490 3610 **e-mail:** katnip@lifedn22.demon.co.uk

Contact: Michael Roberts

Health authority: East London and City

Life Education Centre

The centre works with children and young people in their formative years (3–15) to help them develop an awareness of themselves, the human body, how it functions, and how and why it is affected by substances that upset its delicate equilibrium. They learn to appreciate the physical, mental and emotional effects of substance abuse on the human body, as well as its adverse social effects.

Contact: Michelle Roe

Tel: 0171 600 6969

Funders: Trust grants; statutory

Target age groups: 3–15

Target groups: Parents; community groups; rural communities

Methods and evaluation: The methods used are a mixture of audio-visual, videotape, models, puppets, and teacher-prompted discussion. The style is positive and non-judgemental, allowing young people to make their own decisions about any negative influences that impede their development to their fullest potential.

The project is evaluated internationally by staff, participants and a limited third party evaluation.

It takes the form of a questionnaire in the UK, and some longitudinal research in Australia and the US.

THE MAZE PROJECT

15 Old Ford Road, Bethnal Green, London E2 9PJ

Tel: 0181 983 4782

Contact: Rio Vella

Health authority: East London and City

Other drug services: Training; parents'/carers' drug awareness training

Detached youth work

The initiative provides a youth work service for Tower Hamlets' young people, and supports the project's brief of education prevention to young people who may not be utilising mainstream youth provision.

Contact: Patricia Mata

Tel: 0181 983 4782

Funders: Tudor Trust; Health Authority, London Borough of Tower Hamlets

Needs assessment methods: The need for this initiative came from a community survey, managers' reports to management committee, and pilot studies.

Target age groups: 11 and over

Target groups: Parents; friends of drug users

Methods and evaluation: The initiative uses one-to-one work, as well as group work ouitside the Maze Project base on the street and in and around youth and community centres.

Evaluation is by service users' evaluations; staff cumulative evaluations, manager and management committee evaluations; and performance indicators.

Drug education/prevention work

The work involves basic drug education and teaching on the effects and dangers of drugs, peer group pressure, and harm reduction.

Contacts: Rio Vella, Patricia Mata

Tel: 0181 983 4782

Partner: Network

Funders: Tudor Trust; Health Authority, London Borough of Tower Hamlets; mainstream grants

Needs assessment methods: A working party realised, through community concerns, the need for education/prevention work.

Target age groups: 11 and over

Target group: Parents

Methods and evaluation: Various methods are employed, including group work, community development and support groups and helplines. There is a slide projector for teachers of parents' sessions, youth workers, community groups, and a briefcase containing samples of drugs to show to young people.

Monthly evaluations are by the staff and management committee, local people, professionals and other interested parties, and users of the service. There are also yearly reports and AGMs, and community concerns are highlighted and responded to.

The Maze Café Youth Provision

This is a drop-in youth facility for young people about 14–18 years, running general youth work, support programmes and drug education prevention work.

Contact: Rio Vella

Tel: 0181 983 4782

Partners: Youth and Community Education; London Borough of Tower Hamlets

Funders: London Borough of Tower Hamlets; YWCA

Needs assessment methods: A need for the facility was identified through a local community survey and detached youth worker reports.

Target age groups: 14–18

Target groups: Not at school; neighbourhoods

Methods and evaluation: The facility supports social education for the youth group, and responds to the group's needs as they arise. It provides workshops of informal educational sessions to support the holistic nature of the aims of the project. There are no pool tables or table tennis tables, and youth workers are 'available', not oppressively present.

Cumulative evaluation is by workers, a management committee, daily recordings by youth workers, and sessions statements by the youth group.

METROPOLITAN POLICE YOUTH AND COMMUNITY SECTION (YACS)

Bow Road Police Station, 111 Bow Road, London E3 2AN

Tel: 0181 217 4963   **Fax:** 0181 217 4960

Contact: Adrian Haughton

Health authority: East London and City

Drug awareness/prevention

The initiative explains what a drug is and the destructive effects of drug taking, e.g. criminal involvement; possible addiction; injury and even death; and effects on friends, family and the wider community.

Contact: Les Samways

Tel: 0181 217 4963

Funders: Metropolitan Police

Target age groups: 11 and over

Target groups: Offenders; parents (PTAs); community groups (when requested)

Methods and evaluation: The initiative uses slides to explain and show how some of the most common drugs, e.g. cannabis, cocaine and heroin, are produced and taken, and the effects they can have both physically and mentally.

Evaluation is through questionnaires and staff meetings.

PROJECT LSD (LITERATURE AND SERVICES ON DRUGS)

131 Aberdeen House, 22–24 Highbury Grove, London N5 2EA

Tel: 0171 288 1500   **Fax:** 0171 288 1111

Contacts: Kate Baker/Ilya Varty

Health authority: Camden and Islington

Other drug services: Training; research into lesbian, gay and bisexual drug use and needs.

Detached work in lesbian and gay clubs

The aim of the work is to provide information on drugs, drug use, the effects of drugs, and drug services, and to provide safer sex kits and information, thus enabling individuals to make their own informed decisions.

Contacts: Kate Baker, Ilya Varty

Tel: 0171 288 1500

Partners: Metro-Trust; Naz Project; other safer sex projects

Funders: District Health Authority; charities and trusts

Needs assessment methods: Self-determined questionnaires, distributed in lesbian and gay venues, were used to research drug use patterns, and where lesbians, gays and bisexuals wanted to access services. The results showed high levels of experimental and recreational drug use, and so detached services in lesbian, gay and bisexual venues, as well as information in newspapers became a priority.

Target age group: over 21

Target groups: Lesbians; gays; bisexuals

Methods and evaluation: The work uses trained volunteers to run a stall in the club (with the co-operation of the owner/manager), and to act as peer educators. The stall is bright and attractive, with free condoms, gloves, dams, lube, sweeties, etc. Individuals are free to come to the stall and get written information or to chat. Action-based research is always conducted at these events.

Action-based research has self-determined the evaluation of the work. LSD collates the service user and venue details.

Detached work in lesbian and gay pubs

The aim of the work is to provide information on drugs, drug use, the effects of drugs, and drugs and safer sex services. It also provides safer sex kits, and information on drug use and safer sex.

Contacts: Kate Baker, Ilya Varty

Tel: 0171 288 1500

Partners: Metro-Trust; Naz Project; other safer sex projects

Funders: District Health Authority; charities and trusts; lesbian and gay pubs

Needs assessment methods: Self-determined questionnaires, distributed in lesbian and gay venues, were used to research drug use, patterns, and where lesbians, gays and bisexuals wanted to access services.

Target groups: Lesbians; gays; bisexuals

Methods: The work uses performance pieces and quizzes, with prizes in association with the Project LSD drugs information stall.

Workshops in gay youth groups in London

The workshops aim to improve knowledge of commonly used drugs and their effects, and to improve harm minimisation and negotiation skills around drug use and safer sex.

Contacts: Kate Baker, Ilya Varty

Tel: 0171 288 1500

Funders: London Health Authorities; charities and trusts

Target age groups: 11 and over

Target groups: Lesbians; gays; bisexuals

Methods and evaluation: The workshops use structured sessions and various training/education methods, as well as facilitated discussion, small group working, quizzes, education games and videos.

Participants fill in detailed feedback sheets; completed activities are monitored; and the information is collated and evaluated for the staff, funders and other organisations.

ROYAL BOROUGH OF KENSINGTON AND CHELSEA COMMUNITY EDUCATION

The Town Hall, Horton Street, London W8 7NX

Tel: 0171 361 2980   **Fax:** 0171 937 0038

Contact: Rob Kiteley

Health authority: Kensington and Chelsea

Other drug services: Community safety; training

Drug Action Movement (DAM)

The movement works with young people to provide opportunities to prevent drug misuse.

Contact: Rob Kiteley

Tel: 0171 361 2980

Partners: Youth service; Drug Action Team; Social Services

Funders: Kensington and Chelsea council and sponsors

Needs assessment methods: A survey was carried out called 'Research project to update the facts about young people and their drug use in the Royal Borough 1996'.

Target age groups: 11 and over

Target group: Neighbourhoods

Methods and evaluation: The launch of the Drug Action Team action plan was held in a local nightclub. Young people designed T-shirts, arranged sponsorship, and invited local media personalities. The event used pirate radio jingles (previously used on air) to promote drug awareness.

Forum meetings are held with participants to review arrangements, etc., and Drug Action Teams meet to review what has been achieved.

SOUTHAMPTON WAY YOUTH PROJECT

60 Stanswood Gardens, Sedgmoor Place, Southampton Way, London SE5 7SR

Tel: 0171 701 9022

Contact: Abena Appiah

Health authority: Lambeth, Southwark and Lewisham

Other drug services: Community safety

Main business: To strengthen community relations in the Southampton Way area

Creativity

These projects enable young people to recognise skills that they may be unaware of through activities such as painting, weaving and drawing, etc. The project ran until September 1996.

Contact: Abena Appiah

Tel: 0171 701 9022

Target groups: Community groups (in Southampton Way area)

Methods: There are several methods used by the project: holding discussions, which appears to be a powerful tool for gathering information from the young people on how they feel about living on an estate, and the problems they encounter; asking the youth to discuss or create an image which comes to mind when the word 'drugs' is heard; going on walkabouts in the area to find out what can be provided or removed to improve the area for residents.

Young People At Risk from Drugs

Aims to: ascertain young people's views about living on a particular estate and their knowledge of drugs, as well as any associations made with school on this issue; to give young people a chance to express their views while making them aware of the negative aspects of drug taking (death, homelessness, crime, etc.).

Contact: Abena Appiah

Tel: 0171 701 9022

Funders: Young People at Risk from Drugs (DoH grant scheme); Southampton Way Tenants and Residents Association

Needs assessment methods: A questionnaire was the chosen tool, but as they were filled in quite badly, not much information could be gathered. In response to this, group discussions were used instead.

Target groups: Community groups (in Southampton Way area)

Methods and evaluation: Videos are shown on the effect drugs have on people, and leaflets are distributed. Young people are encouraged to write articles for the estate newsletter, which is distributed on a regular basis, and promotes environmental awareness, and emphasises the need to respect the area in which you live. Equal opportunities principles are outlined, in an attempt to get young people to respect all those with whom they come into contact.

Evaluation methods include: attendance record; session recordings; feedback from young people. Also, regular observations of participants to identify change in: communication with both adults and peers; participation; or contribution to any project work.

YAP (YOUTH AWARENESS PROGRAMME) TOTTENHAM

Selby Centre, Selby Road, Tottenham, London N17 8JN

Tel: 0181 493 9000   **Fax:** 0181 493 9279

Contact: Jib

Health authority: Enfield and Haringey

Other drug services: Treatment; training

Danny Role-play

The role-play allows the group to experience the situation of a young person who gets into debt and shows what they would do.

Contact: Aurangzeb Khaliq

Tel: 0181 493 9000

Funders: Young People at Risk from Drugs (DoH grant scheme)

Needs assessment methods: Research was carried out in field studies, schools, colleges, youth centres, and client case notes.

Target age groups: 11–21

Target groups: Offenders; black Caribbean; black African; other minority ethnic groups; children in care

Methods and evaluation: The case study is presented to the group using role-play and involving members of the class (volunteers). After the case study, the group are asked to list ideas on how the young person can get out of the situation. The class then discusses the ideas to see if they are feasible or not.

Evaluation is carried out by the Home Office, Her Majesty's Inspectors (OFSTED), and the Policy Studies Institute, and takes the form of questionnaires, observations, group discussions, and supervision.

Question and Answers

The project aims to provide drugs information, covering the effects and harm minimisation, in a non-judgemental way and in a confidential environment.

Contact: Aurangzeb Khaliq

Tel: 0181 493 9000

Funders: Young People at Risk from Drugs; Health Authority

Needs assessment methods: Questionnaires were carried out in informal situations such as field studies, schools, colleges, and youth clubs. Notes from clients' case studies were also involved.

Target age groups: 11 and over

Target groups: Offenders; black Caribbean; black African; other ethnic groups; children in care

Methods and evaluation: After an initial introduction, the group are asked to call out all the drugs that they have heard of. These are listed on the board and the group are asked to choose a drug for discussion. The facilitator asks the group what they know about the drug and corrects any misinformation.

Evaluation is carried out by the Home Office, Her Majesty's Inspectors (OFSTED), and the Policy Studies Institute, and takes the form of questionnaires, observations, group discussions, and supervision.

Greater Manchester

SALFORD COMMUNITY DRUG ADVISORY SERVICE

1st Floor, 1 King Street, Eccles, Manchester M30 DAE

Tel: 0161 787 7343   **Fax:** 0161 789 0360

Contact: Peter Polese

Health authority: Salford and Trafford

Other drug services: Treatment; community safety; criminal justice, training

---

Specialist outreach worker for young people

The outreach worker can maximise contact with young drug users who are not in contact with any services, thereby assisting in the treatment, education and prevention of drug misuse in Salford.

Contact: Kath Bennett

Tel: 0161 207 7188

Funder: Salford Social Services

Needs assessment methods: The need for an outreach worker was highlighted by *Young people's drug use in Salford,* which was published in January 1995, as well as in-depth semi-structured interviews, and self-completed questionnaires.

Target age groups: 11 and over

Target groups: Offenders; children in care; parents (support groups); neighbourhoods; community groups (Little Hulton)

Methods and evaluation: The outreach worker is responsible for the following projects: quizzes on drugs, poster project/competition, and young women's groups. Outreach activities include parents' evenings, individual counselling, and youth clubs.

DASH (DRUG ADVICE AND SUPPORT IN HULME)

Zion Community Centre, Zion Crescent, Hulme, Manchester M15 5BY

Tel: 0161 226 0202   **Fax:** 0161 227 9862

Contact: Sarah Higson

Health authority: Manchester

Other drug services: Treatment; training

Outreach work

The outreach work targets young black people in Moss Side with information, advice and support around drugs and HIV. This initiative ran until April 1996.

Contact: Denise Williams

Tel: 0161 226 0202

Funders: Manchester Health Authority

Needs assessment methods: Informal discussions revealed a lack of targeted information, a lack of black workers, and a lack of access to mainstream services – seen as 'white', and not appropriate.

Target groups: Black Caribbean; black African; neighbourhoods

Methods: The work uses many different methods including: provision of leaflets and verbal information and support; a 'gateway' to other services through befriending; and group work in schools, etc., with more formalised drug education. A poster devised and produced with relevance to the Moss Side black community, and the community radio station was used to give out information. A black worker from the community serves as an effective peer educator.

LIFELINE

101–103 Oldham Street, Manchester M4 1LW

Tel: 0161 839 2054   **Fax:** 0161 834 5903 **e-mail:** drughelp@lifeline.demon.co.uk

Health authority: Manchester

Other drug services: Treatment; community safety; criminal justice; training; specialist services include: Lifeline for parents, family work, safer dancing campaign

Safer Dancing Campaign

This aims to provide information about recreational drugs to young people, mainly in a nightclub setting that incorporates a number of strategies aimed at reducing drug-related harm.

Contact: Natalie Melton

Tel: 0161 839 2054

Partners: Manchester City Council; Manchester Drug Prevention Initiative; police; local nightclubs; nightclub promoters

Funders: Manchester City Council

Target age groups: 11 and over

Target groups: Users of dance drugs

Methods and evaluation: Much of the work is based on the exchange of information between staff/volunteers, club promoters and young drug users in an informal setting. This has involved a number of steering groups and drug users in developing methods of providing information and advice; they have been trained to provide others with advice, and have helped develop policies for nightclubs to reduce risks for young people.

There was a written evaluation of some of the gender-specific materials which was carried out by an outside researcher. It also included a questionnaire for young women and the drugs workers.

NACRO (NATIONAL ASSOCIATION FOR THE CARE AND RESETTLEMENT OF OFFENDERS) – HOUSING IN GREATER MANCHESTER

NACRO, 1 Rosina Street, Openshaw, Manchester M11 1HX

Tel: 0161 301 1946

Contact: Lesley Steel

Health authority: Manchester

Other drug services: Community safety; criminal justice; training; supported accommodation

Counselling and group work

These sessions allow residents to explore alternative positive lifestyle changes in a supported environment. Examples of topics covered are: harm reduction, healthy lifestyles, first-aid training, relaxation techniques, and services available in the community.

Contact: Lesley Steel

Tel: 0161 301 1946

Partner: Greater Manchester Probation Service

Funders: Greater Manchester Probation Service; Local Authority; National Lottery Charities Board; charity

Needs assessment methods: Probation research indicated that 70 per cent of their clients had drug problems.

Target age groups: 11 and over

Target groups: Offenders; males; homeless

Methods and evaluation: Information is given to all residents about local drug services, and written information is also available. Groupwork sessions cover harm reduction and all aspects of drug use; methods used include: general discussion, drugs card game, videos, and role-play. Groupwork sessions also include basic living skills, budgeting and health issues. Residents also have access to training courses, e.g. first-aid, equal opportunities, basic maintenance, as well as an opportunity to gain NVQ qualifications in core skills.

Evaluation is through monitoring of specific targets, interviews with staff, written evaluation by reviewing agencies on the progress of their client. Independent research was also carried out on behalf of the Department of Health.

NEWTON HEATH YOUTH AND COMMUNITY ASSOCIATION

2 Bilsland Walk, Newton Heath, Manchester M40 1LW

Tel: 0161 681 6270

Contact: Anne Catherine Bowles

Health authority: Manchester

Other drug services: Community safety; training

Main business: Youth and community work activities

Drugs prevention initiative

The aims of the initiative are: to increase awareness of the risks associated with drug misuse and engage young people in structured activities; to increase their involvement in the young people's forum; to support local residents and parents by providing information.

Contact: Anne Catherine Bowles

Tel: 0161 681 6270

Partner: East Manchester Community Forum

Funders: Home Office Drug Prevention Initiative; City Council, East Manchester Community Forum support

Needs assessment methods: A survey of young people highlighted the high drug use in the area and very little help, support and advice available to the users and their families.

Target groups: Offenders; parents; tenants group; volunteers

Methods: The sessional worker is engaging young people in sport and activities, assessing their needs and attitudes, developing a local drug information resource and promoting its use. Local residents and parents are offered support in their roles, as well as help, information, training and advice. Outreach work takes place on a sessional basis, two or three nights a week, delivering drug awareness and group/peer support, and encouraging young people to become involved in the youth and community association and the young people's forum.

SAFE IN THE CITY

354 Waterloo Road, Northenden, Greater Manchester M8 9AB

Tel: 0161 740 4183   **Fax:** 0161 795 7152

Contact: Mark Lee, Carol Smith

Health authority: Manchester

Main business: Outreach – to make contact and offer support to estranged, marginalised young people who live on or hang around the streets of Manchester. It is a street-based project.

Streetwork

This street-based project offers support, advice, advocacy and mediation to young people who are estranged or marginalised from caring adult support networks.

Contact: Mark Lee, Carol Smith

Tel: 0161 740 4183

Funder: The Children's Society

Needs assessment methods: Outreach, street-walks, contacts, research.

Target age group: 11–16

Target groups: Homeless; neighbourhoods

Methods and evaluation: The work includes street work, street-walks, core time (guaranteed to be at a certain place, at a certain time, on a certain day), discussions, counselling, mediation, advice, advocacy, and support.

Evaluation is by inspections and questionnaires.

GREATER MANCHESTER POLICE – OPERATION JIGSAW

Park Lane Police Station, Bury New Road, Higher Broughton, Salford, Greater Manchester M7 0LG

Tel: 0161 856 5162   **Fax:** 0161 856 5162

Contact: Frank Doyle

Health authority: Manchester

Other drug services: Community safety; criminal justice; training

Jiggo 96

Initiatives were held to divert young people into sporting activities in May 1996.

Contact: Alan Brown

Tel: 0161 856 5162

Partners: Manchester County Football Association; UEFA

Funder: Manchester County Football Association

Target age groups: 11–21

Methods and evaluation: A football competition for teams of 8, run by the Manchester County Football Association, was supported by literature provided by the police, including *Sport – a real habit*, a factual guide to drugs, parents' guide, etc. The finals were held at Manchester United Football Club's stadium as pre-match entertainment before the Euro 96 matches.

999 Challenge

Groups of 20 youths attended a 12-week programme – 4 weeks police, 4 weeks ambulance, 4 weeks fire brigade (one night per week) – culminating in a 999 Challenge Day, where they were tested on what they had learned by dealing with an emergency scenario. The project ran from May to September 1996.

Contact: Phil Gleave

Tel: 0161 856 5162

Partners: Fire brigade; ambulance service

Funders: Police, fire and ambulance services

Target age groups: 11–18

Target group: Offenders

Methods: The groups were drawn from various areas covered by the force, and attended four evenings with the police for input on police procedures and drug issues. Points were awarded for attendance, with extra points for community work. The Challenge Day consisted of a series of practical exercises, and the winning team was the one that amassed the most points over both the 12-week period and the Challenge Day.

MANCUNIAN HEALTH PROMOTION SPECIALIST SERVICE

Health Promotion Service, Withington Hospital, Nell Lane, West Didsbury, Greater Manchester M20 2LR

Tel: 0161 291 3641   **Fax:** 0161 291 3643

Contact: Janet Mantle

Health authority: Manchester

Other drug services: Training

Raising children in a drug-using society

This is a 10-week accredited course to support parents in working and communicating with children about drug issues.

Contact: Janet Mantle

Tel: 0161 291 3641

Funders: Manchester Health Authority; Marks & Spencer

Needs assessment methods: The need for the course was identified via feedback from the Healthy Schools Award.

Target groups: Parents; neighbourhoods

Methods and evaluation: This 10-week accredited course is for parents to improve their communication and assertiveness skills and their knowledge of parenting skills and drugs, in order to help them cope with drug-using children or children's enquiries regarding drugs. The course also involves group work, discussion, project work, and input from specialist workers.

The course is evaluated by staff and participants through surveys, discussions and self-assessment of progress, as well as a longer-term follow-up. It is also accredited by the Open College (Manchester).

Merseyside

PADA (PARENTS AGAINST DRUG ABUSE) WIRRAL

The Roundabout Centre, 1 Stanley Road, Birkenhead, Merseyside L41 7BG

Tel: 0151 652 9108

Contact: Joan Keogh

Health authority: Wirral

Annual parents' convention

The convention aims to encourage parents and concerned citizens around the UK: to start up groups in their own areas; to work in their communities towards demand reduction; to set up drop-in centres; and to educate parents and children about the dangers of drug use.

Contact: Joan Keogh

Tel: 0151 652 9108

Funders: Birkenhead Lions, Merseyside Drug Prevention Team; attending parents; PADA

Needs assessment methods: The need for the convention was highlighted by attending a government sponsored conference in conjunction with Lifeline and ADFAM; and through listening to complaints by parents that the conference was not what they wanted, and then following this up by finding out what was needed.

Target groups: Parents; community groups; rural communities

Evaluation: Evaluation forms are given to each participant at the convention.

Duke of Westminster's Award Scheme

The main focus of the scheme is to encourage young people to become involved in drug awareness and prevention.

Contact: Joan Keogh

Tel: 0151 652 9108

Funders: PADA; Birkenhead Lions

Target age groups: 11–18

Target groups: Community groups

Methods and evaluation: The particular activities are left to the young people to decide upon, as this project is an award scheme. The winners receive a silver cup and plaque, and a cheque of £500 towards their project.

Evaluation is carried out by PADA's management committee and those involved in setting up the various projects, and takes the form of noting the number of participants who enter for the award scheme.

General duties of PADA

These include drugs awareness, education and prevention for parents and families.

Contact: Joan Keogh

Tel: 0151 652 9108

Funders: Various charities

Target groups: Parents; neighbourhoods; community groups; rural communities

Methods: PADA has a drop-in centre, makes home visits, and gives talks to groups both in the Wirral and around the country. It encourages parents to start up their own groups around the country.

PADA awareness day

This is a day held to show school-aged children that they can enjoy themselves without the use of drugs. It took place in October 1996, and it is hoped that it can be made a regular event.

Contact: Ken Fretwell

Tel: 0151 652 9108

Partners: Education; police; youth service

Funder: PADA

SHADO (SUPPORTIVE HELP AND DEVELOPMENT ORGANISATION LTD)

Family Support Centre, 120 Stonebridge Lane, Croxteth, Liverpool, Merseyside L11 9AZ

Tel: 0151 546 1141   **Fax:** 0151 548 6972

Contact: Audrey Brooks

Health authority: Liverpool

Other drug services: Treatment; community safety; training

Main business: Emotional counselling and support

Awareness programme for young people

The programme works to provide young people with relevant, up-to-date, supportive help and information around drugs, solvents, HIV and related health and social issues.

Contact: Pauline O'Keeffe

Tel: 0151 546 1141

Funders: Health Authority; charitable source

Target age groups: 11 and over

Target groups: Offenders; community groups

Methods: The programme provides up-to-date, relevant information for young people, including support and/or counselling. Peer education programmes are also run at SHADO and other organisations as well as youth health groups which include work around drugs/alcohol, etc.

Detached outreach project

The project aims to work with young people on the streets or where they are to be found, and to provide information, advice and support. It also involves young people in sport, and social and creative activities. The project finished in December 1996.

Contact: Audrey Brooks

Tel: 0151 546 1141

Funder: Charitable source

Target age groups: 11 and over

Target groups: Offenders; not at school; homeless; children in care; parents; community organisations

Methods: This project offers good youth work practice on the streets offering relevant information/support and advice; working closely with other workers in the area; and working with sports centres and other appropriate contacts.

Young persons' daily drop-in

SHADO works with young people (11 years and over) to provide a daily supportive, safe environment for young people to meet, especially as schools are now on continental hours. Many young people bring their problems, some have experimented with drugs.

Contact: Bill McIntyre

Tel: 0151 546 1141

Funder: Charitable funder

Needs assessment methods: There was no formal assessment, but before the young persons' drop-in time was set up, young people dropped into the agency all through the day.

There was a very obvious need to have a place/time set aside.

Target age groups: 11 and over

Target groups: Not at school; homeless; children in care; parents

Methods: SHADO aims to: provide a supportive, safe environment, in which young people can meet and talk, which is not a youth club; work with and complement youth work in the area; give information and advice in a group or on an individual basis, with counselling available as appropriate. At the same time, health awareness and peer education is promoted.

HEALTH LINE PROJECT

88 Sheil Road, Liverpool, Merseyside L6 3AF

Tel: 0151 263 0557   **Fax:** 0151 260 4747

Contact: Paulene Warnock

Health authority: Liverpool

Other drug services: Training; health education

Main business: Delivers health education programmes

Work with young people around drugs information

The aim of the work is: to provide young people with accurate information about drugs, their use and their effect; to explore their attitudes to drug use; and to develop skills which enable them to make informed choices about their own involvement in drug use.

Contact: Paulene Warnock

Tel: 0151 263 0557

Partners: Liverpool Youth Service; Youth and Community; Roscommon School

Funders: Liverpool Health Authority; Liverpool City Council; Local Education Authority; youth service

Target age groups: 11 and over

Target group: Neighbourhoods

Methods and evaluation: The youth service's delivery of education depends on the relationship developed between young people and youth workers. Work around drugs issues is delivered in response to the needs identified in negotiations between the worker and young people, and in response to spontaneous interest.

To evaluate the work, youth workers keep records of sessions and work to a development plan. Outcomes are measured against objectives set in the plan, and also against individual session plans.

HIT

Cavern Walks, 8 Matthew Street, Liverpool, Merseyside L2 6RE

Tel: 0151 227 4012   **Fax:** 0151 227 4023   **e-mail:** hit@hit1.demon.co.uk

Contact: Andrew M Bennett

Health authority: Liverpool

Other drug services: Training

Wirral City Lands Drug Information Campaign

The project involved the delivery of drug information messages involving multi-component media: 3D leaflets and posters, training courses for parents, murals, and community events. The project finished in December 1996.

Contact: Andrew M Bennett

Tel: 0151 227 4012

Partners: Drug Prevention Team; Wirral City Lands

Funders: Wirral City Lands; Merseyside Drug Prevention Initiative

Needs assessment methods: Discussions were held with local community members as well as pre-campaign interviews with the target group (11–14-year-olds) and parents.

Target age groups: 11–14

Target group: Parents

Methods and evaluation: The project carried out research before the campaign and produced materials, including 3-D cards and posters which were distributed. They also used murals, competitions and personal appearances by Harry Hammond.

The evaluator, Sheila Henderson, was commissioned by Merseyside Drug Prevention Initiative. The evaluation, carried out from January to April 1997, took the form of interviews with focus groups pre- and post-campaign.

SEFTON YOUTH SERVICE

Birkdale Youth Centre, Windy Harbour Road, Southport, Merseyside PR8 3DT

Tel: 01704 579836

Contact: Thelma Cooper

Health authority: Southport and Formby

Main business: Social education of young people to help with their transition to adulthood

mobi-Woodvale: mobile information centre

The mobile aims: to provide information and support to enable young people to make informed choices on drugs and health issues; to offer stimulating activities, such as stock-car racing, climbing, Duke of Edinburgh's awards; and to encourage young people's involvement in the community.

Contacts: Thelma Cooper, Dave Law

Tel: 0151 934 4878

Partners: Merseyside Drugs Council; local training schemes; Woodvale Community Centre

Funders: Home Office; Sefton Youth Service

Target age groups: 11–21

Target groups: Not at school; neighbourhoods

Methods and evaluation: Workers on the mobile information centre (a converted social services ambulance) work in pairs running groupwork sessions, educational games and videos. Follow-up activities and community projects are planned with the young people.

There is an ongoing evaluation, with a full evaluation after 12 months.

TRANMERE COMMUNITY PROJECT

Whitfield Street, Tranmere, Wirral, Merseyside L42 0LG

Tel: 0151 649 8017   **Fax:** 0151 647 4845

Contact: Gill Quayle

Health authority: Wirral

Main business: To provide community education, employment advice and a social centre (coffee bar)

Substance abuse project

The project involves outreach and youth work with young people in the area who abuse or are at risk of abusing drugs (especially alcohol).

Contact: Wendy Robertson

Tel: 0151 649 8017

Funders: Merseyside Drug Prevention Team; Rank Foundation; Health Authority

Needs assessment methods: A questionnaire was distributed to the community. The response reflected a knowledge of attitudes to drugs, and also gave feedback on how to tackle any drug-related problems.

Target age groups: 11–18

Target group: Neighbourhoods

Methods: The project used various methods: outreach – street work, meeting and talking with young people; giving out information and referring to other agencies; using the centre as a base for longer-term projects, e.g. summer programme; schools work – running lessons about drug awareness with pupils; and working around the school at lunchtimes, when workers are available to talk and give information.

Middlesex

RICHMOND DRUG EDUCATION PROJECT – WHAT'S THE SCORE?

Hampton Youth Project, 32 Tangley Park Road, Hampton, Middlesex TW12 3YH

Tel: 0181 941 9566

Contact: Alison Hopgood

Health authority: Kingston and Richmond

Other drug services: Training; drug training for full-time/part-time voluntary staff

Detached street work

The aim of the work is to raise young people's awareness of the risks of drug use, especially those who are not in contact with the youth service or other youth groups, and to provide information on harm minimisation.

Contact: Richard Campbell

Tel: 0181 941 9566

Funders: Local charities; Health Promotion Unit/Service

Needs assessment methods: a survey by the Community Drug and Alcohol Team on drug use in the borough highlighted the fact that no detached provision was available at that time.

Target age groups: 11–18

Methods and evaluation: There are many different methods used: approaching young people in the street, in parks and on estates, and engaging with them; giving out leaflets on drugs, and stimulating conversations on drugs and health; distributing condoms; building relationships; and trying to get young people involved in work on photostories and other projects. Workers operate in a pair – male/female, 1 full-time, 1 part-time – in a non-judgemental, confidential way, and give out cards with a number for young people to call if they want any information on drugs.

The youth service has developed an evaluation model, which it applies to the work. The various methods include: assessing the numbers of people contacted and recontacted, and anecdotal evidence of change in knowledge, attitude and behaviour. A dictaphone is used to record immediately and each session is written up afterwards. This is collated in a bi-annual report.

Drug awareness workshops

Workshops are run in clubs, colleges and schools, and explore drug information, attitudes to drugs, why people use drugs and making decisions about drug use.

Contact: Richard Campbell

Tel: 0181 941 9566

Funders: Local charities; Health Promotion Unit/Service

Needs assessment methods: There was feedback from club workers on young people's levels of knowledge and their activity around drugs.

Methods and evaluation: These are informal workshops that look at drug facts using games, flipcharts, and group work; attitudes to drugs, using games, flipcharts, group discussions; and why young people use/abuse drugs (including, assessing risks and making choices). Workshops are individually tailored to take account of age and group make-up.

Each participant fills in an evaluation form. The worker evaluates each session and collates information. Questions include: Was the workshop fun? Did it make you more aware? What else would you like to see? Was it boring? Do you feel more able to make informed decisions about your drug use? The worker notes any comments and responses.

Outreach work

This involves non-structured work in clubs and colleges.

Contact: Richard Campbell

Tel: 0181 941 9566

Funders: Local charities; Health Promotion Unit/Service

Methods: This very informal approach involves taking information into a club or college, leaving it around for young people to see, then trying to promote discussion, talking one-to-one and in groups, and getting young people to talk about their own drug use in a confidential and non-judgemental environment.

Peer education project

The project aimed to give a number of young people the opportunity to look at themselves and drug use, society and drug use, and themselves and society, and at what provisions they feel should be available. Participants also analysed the effectiveness of peer education. The project ran until December 1996.

Contact: Richard Campbell

Tel: 0181 941 9566

Funder: Drug project

Needs assessment methods: A need was identified by drug awareness workers to look at the reality of drugs in our society.

Methods: The training on this project involves 12 sessions, one of which is residential. The sessions are: Getting to know each other; Basic drug awareness; Attitudes to drugs; Residential; Drug agencies/treatments; Visiting agencies/clients; Putting it together; Drugs and the media; Drugs and the law; Debate on drugs – guest speakers; Implications of debate; Where am I now?; Where do we go from here?

There is also an assessment of peer education and an evaluation procedure.

BRENT AND HARROW HEALTH PROMOTION UNIT

Grace Ward, Northwick Park and St Marks, Watford Road, Harrow, Middlesex HA1 3UJ

Tel: 0181 869 3643   **Fax:** 0181 869 3641

Contacts: Paul O'Sullivan/Tim Walsh

Health authority: Brent and Harrow

Other drug services: Training; policy departments for schools

Main business: Health promotion: provider development

Drugs education evening for parents

Through this initiative, schools in Harrow and Brent can have evening sessions for parents/governors tailor-made to their needs.

Contact: Lesley de Meza

Tel: 0181 869 3643

Partners: Harrow Advisory Teachers; Brent Grants for Education Support and Training Drugs Project; Metropolitan Police; local drugs agencies

Funders: Harrow Advisory Teachers, Brent Grants for Education Support and Training Drugs Project; police; drug agencies

Target group: Parents

Methods and evaluation: Typically, an expert gives a talk (10–40 mins), then parents go into workshop groups. Quizzes, discussion and videos are sometimes used, depending on the school.

Sometimes a 'Drugs: a family matter' evaluation form is used; otherwise it is a standard questionnaire.

You want to know the truth about drugs

This project involves researching, writing and illustrating a booklet, *You want to know the truth about drugs*, for young people. It is aimed at harm reduction, and possibly drugs prevention education, and contains information on local services.

Contact: Lesley de Meza

Tel: 0181 869 3643

Partners: Advisory teachers in Harrow; Brent East Drugs Project Co-ordinator; local drugs agencies; local sexual health and drugs teams

Funder: Health Authority

Needs assessment methods: Confidential questionnaires; discussion workshops; drama workshops; and content, style, layout, and illustration discussions were used to establish young people's needs/wants.

Target age groups: 11–21

Target groups: Not at school; homeless; children in care

Evaluation: All involved were invited to comment on drafts of the booklet. Alterations were made as necessary.

SUBSTANCE MISUSE MANAGEMENT PROJECT

Grace House, Harrovian Business Village, Bessborough Road, Harrow, Middlesex HA1 3EX

Tel: 0181 966 1109   **Fax:** 0181 423 7314

Contact: David Sheehan

Health authority: Brent and Harrow

Other drug services: Treatment; training; payment and support for GPs to treat drug users; development of local shared care

Youth advice service

The aims are: to develop youth advice services in primary care settings; to involve and develop a role for the Primary Health Care Team and GPs; to pilot a range of methods for targeting young people and appropriate interventions; to promote drugs and sexual health issues amongst young people.

Contact: Jean Claude Barjolin

Tel: 0181 966 1109

Partners: Substance Misuse Management Project; Health Authority

Funder: Health Authority

Needs assessment methods: Interviews were held with GPs and Primary Health Care Team staff, and with youth groups and peer education group.

Target age groups: 11 and over

Target group: Neighbourhoods

Methods: The service takes the form of an informal walk-in/drop-in at centres. It is not promoted as specific to drugs, but as covering any area of concern, with information materials appropriate to young people. There is outreach to local groups, and letters of invitation are sent to young people via GP lists.

TURNING POINT (HOUNSLOW)

8 Pownall Gardens, Hounslow, Middlesex TW3 1YW

Tel: 0181 577 3294   **Fax:** 0181 814 0717

Contact: Neerja Kapoor

Health authority: Ealing, Hammersmith and Hounslow

Other drug services: Criminal justice; training; in the process of setting up an arrest referral scheme

Community outreach service

The service provides one-to-one information about harm minimisation, acupuncture and needle exchange. The aim is to make contact with those who are potentially at risk from drug use, and who are not in contact with any other agencies. Apart from this work with clients, the outreach service provides training to professionals, and education and prevention sessions to those at risk.

Contact: Neerja Kapoor

Tel: 0181 577 3294

Partners: Corporate HIV unit; youth and community

Funders: Department of Health; Social Services

Methods and evaluation: Outreach workers work on a one-to-one basis with clients around safer drug use and safer injecting. For those clients who are modifying their drug use, support and information are provided about how to do this safely, as well as acupuncture sessions. For those users who are injecting, clean works can be supplied, although this has to be done very discreetly in outreach settings. Written information is also provided on all of the above in the form of posters and leaflets (in various languages), and the same information is provided over the telephone.

Evaluation is through a presentation to the funders who review the service. The presentation is followed by questions, and follow-up meetings are booked in.

HOUNSLOW YOUTH AND COMMUNITY SERVICE

78 St Johns Road, Isleworth, Middlesex TW7 6RU

Tel: 0181 568 3697   **Fax:** 0181 862 7788

Contact: Yvonne McNamara

Health authority: Ealing, Hammersmith and Hounslow

Other drug services: Community safety; criminal justice; training

Health information project

The project provides drug, alcohol and sexual health services to young people aged 14–25 years

Contact: Yvonne McNamara

Tel: 0181 568 3697

Partners: London Borough of Hounslow; Corporate HIV unit; Ealing, Hammersmith and Hounslow Health Agency

Funders: Ealing, Hammersmith and Hounslow Health Agency; Hounslow Youth and Community Service

Needs assessment methods: A survey regarding drug use was carried out in part of the borough in which 98 per cent of young persons questioned used drugs.

Target age groups: 14–25

Peer theatre-in-education project

The project involves work with young people aged 16–25 years around community safety issues – particularly drug and alcohol misuse. Twelve unemployed young people train in forum theatre, put together a production and tour schools, youth groups, etc.

Contact: Yvonne McNamara

Tel: 0181 568 3697

Partners: European Social Fund; ARTSNET

Funders: European Social Fund; Hounslow Youth and Community Service; ARTSNET

Needs assessment methods: A need for this project came from a formal survey with young people, a local authority survey, a police survey, and informal discussions with young people.

Target age groups: 16–25

Norfolk

NORCAS

11 Parsonage Square, Norwich, Norfolk NR2 1AS

Tel: 01603 767093   **Fax:** 01603 767093

Contact: Penny McVeigh

Health authority: East Norfolk

Other drug services: Treatment; criminal justice; training; shared care with GPs

Drugs and alcohol/young people project

This comprises drug and alcohol projects located in Great Yarmouth, Lowestoft and Thetford.

Contact: Mike Soper

Tel: 01603 767093

Partners: Youth Community Services; Social Services; Local Education Authority

Funders: National Lottery Charities Board; NORCAS funds

Target age groups: 11 and over

Target groups: Not at school; homeless; children in care; rural communities

Methods: The project works closely with youth and the community, and existing NORCAS services, to provide a detached service to young people, equalling their social setting. In 1997, premises are being established, after a needs assessment of young people, by young people, has identified the best resource to be provided.

NORFOLK YOUTH AND COMMUNITY SERVICE

Room 051, County Hall, Norwich, Norfolk NR1 2DL

Tel: 01603 222342   **Fax:** 01603 222119

Contact: Martyn Livermore

Health authority: East Norfolk

Other drug services: Treatment

Information and advice

This covers the provision of drug education information to 13–19-year-olds via interactive computer packages and one-to-one work, as well as training for part-time youth workers.

Contact: Peter Bainbridge

Tel: 01603 766994

Partners: NORCAS; Norwich Gay Men's Health; Community Alcohol and Drugs Service; Matthew Project; Bure Clinic; East Norfolk Health Authority

Funders: Norfolk County Council; East Norfolk Health Authority

Needs assessment methods: A two-year MSc student study from the Cranfield Institute showed the need for quality, up-to-date, peer-led advice and information, as well as referral.

Target age groups: 13–19

Target groups: Neighbourhoods; rural communities

Methods: Training given to new staff.

THE MATTHEW PROJECT

24 Pottersgate, Norwich, Norfolk NR2 1DX

Tel: 01603 626123   **Fax:** 01603 630411   **e-mail:** 106035.2270@compuserve.com

Contact: Peter Farley

Health authority: East Norfolk

Other drug services: Treatment; community safety; criminal justice; training; 24-hour helpline, counselling advice and support

Tackle Express (mobile service)

The service aims to raise awareness of services on offer, to provide information and support, and to build relationships with young people.

Contact: Mark Heybourne

Tel: 01603 626123

Partners: Schools; youth services; police; parish councils; churches

Funders: East Norfolk Health Authority; variety of charitable trusts

Target age groups: 11 and over

Methods and evaluation: Methods include: giving information; practical development; visual arts; music; games; role-play; the Matthew Project outreach caravan; the Matthew Project youth work caravan; and the Young People's Health outreach caravan.

Evaluation is by the Norwich City College Research Department, commissioned by the East Norfolk Health Commission.

Northamptonshire

CAN (COUNCIL ON ADDICTION FOR NORTHAMPTONSHIRE)

81 St Giles Street, Northampton, Northamptonshire NN1 1JF

Tel: 01604 27027   **Fax:** 01604 29577

Contact: Robin Burgess

Health authority: Northamptonshire

Other drug services: Treatment; community safety; criminal justice; training

---

Single Regeneration Budget project – drug outreach

This education/prevention project, in a deprived area of Northampton and in Corby, aims at early intervention with young people. It also works with schools and community groups.

Contact: Helen Riches

Tel: 01604 27027

Funders: Social Services; Single Regeneration Budget; Northampton Borough Council

Needs assessment methods: Various questionnaires and an area profile were carried out by the Single Regeneration Budget team and the Health Authority. Significant issues about drugs emerged from four of the six areas involved.

Target age groups: 11 and over

Target groups: Not at school; neighbourhoods; community groups

Methods and evaluation: This is a very eclectic project, similar to the Home Office projects.

Youth work

This involves liaison with youth clubs all over the county.

Contact: Single Regeneration Budget worker

Tel: 01604 27027

Funders: Social Services; self-financed

Target age groups: 11 and over

Nottinghamshire

NORTH NOTTS HEALTH PROMOTION UNIT/SERVICE

NNHP, 72 Portland Street, Kirkby-in-Ashfield, Nottinghamshire NG17 7AE

Tel: 01623 751984   **Fax:** 01623 752457

Contacts: Jill Lancaster, Christine Nield

Main business: Health promotion, training, advice and consultation, support and resources on a range of health issues

---

apa (ASSOCIATION FOR THE PREVENTION OF ADDICTION) OPEN DOORS: UNDER 21 SPECIALIST SERVICE

Open Doors, First Floor, 17 Huntingdon Street, Nottingham, Nottinghamshire NG1 3JH

Tel: 01159 243506   **Fax:** 01159 242838

Contact: Sue Loakes

Health authority: Nottingham

Other drug services: Treatment; training

Creative workshops with young people

The workshops enable young people to become involved in creating, designing and co-planning drama workshops, poetry, etc.

Contact: Sue Loakes

Tel: 01159 243506

Target groups: Offenders; homeless; children in care

Drop-in

Drop-in offered three afternoons a week; to provide the possibility for young people to access services quickly, and to meet other young people to access support.

Contact: Sue Loakes

Tel: 01159 243506

Funders: Health Authority; Social Services

Target age groups: 11–21

Target groups: Offenders; not at school; homeless; children in care

COMMUNITY DRUGS PREVENTION PROJECT

TNC, 60 Sneinton Hollows, Sneinton, Nottingham NG2 4AA

Tel: 0115 950 5110

Contact: Jan Dawson

Health authority: Nottingham

Other drug services: Training; work with parents

Family Centre parents group

The group aims to raise the level of parents' knowledge about drugs issues, and to develop their communications skills and self-esteem to enable them to communicate with their children and to cope better should they discover in the future that their children are using drugs.

Contact: Jan Dawson

Tel: 0115 950 5110

Partners: Senior Development Officer; Nottingham Council

Funder: Drugs Prevention Initiative

Target group: Parents

Methods and evaluation: Meetings include: drug quizzes (attitude continuums, brainstorming, discussion); looking at how we feel about ourselves and why; basic level transactional analysis; and improving communication using role-play and case scenarios. Sessional workers are involved for self-esteem raising.

Evaluation is through verbal feedback of participants and facilitators, evaluation forms and group discussion.

Music group

This initiative involves working with young people from different cultures in a recording studio to produce and market a drugs awareness record. Sessions are held on drugs information, cultural differences, attitude, lyrics, technical information, etc.

Contact: Nick Croft

Tel: 0115 950 5110

Partners: Nottingham Black Initiative (NBI); Peer Pressure Records; ACNA Community Centre

Funders: Community Drug Prevention Team; Nottingham City Council

Target groups: Black Caribbean; black African; black other; Indian; Pakistani; Bangladeshi

Methods: Methods evolve through a process of consultation between participating agencies and young people.

DRUG EDUCATION TEAM

College Street Centre, College Street, Nottingham NG3 6AN

Tel: 0115 953 5041   **Fax:** 0115 953 5041

Contact: Paul Mein

Health authority: Nottingham

Act Aware

Performance projects were devised and performed by young people, and supported by professional artists, to give young people an opportunity to express their views and feelings about both legal and illegal drugs, and, through performance, to make their own statement on drug misuse. The projects finished in March 1996.

Contact: Karen Smith

Tel: 0115 95 35041

Partners: Roundabout Theatre in Education company; 'Next Stage' Nottinghamshire Adult Education

Funders: Department for Education and Employment 13b; Nottinghamshire City Council

Methods and evaluation: Members of Roundabout Theatre in Education Company and local professional performers worked with various groups of young people, enabling them to produce their own performance piece on a drug prevention theme. The whole project culminated in a series of performances around the county from 18 to 24 March. There were five main performance strands: A-Level expressive/performing arts students; GCSE drama students; 11th session (out of school arts workshops); Nottinghamshire Adult Education; and Roundabout Theatre in Education Company. Backdrops and settings were provided by two Saturday morning art workshops.

Parents of participants were the evaluators, and questionnaires were used to ascertain how parents and children used the project as a way of talking together on drug-related issues; and how involvement increased their knowledge or altered attitudes.

LIFE EDUCATION CENTRE NOTTINGHAMSHIRE

Police HQ, Sherwood Lodge, Arnold, Nottingham NG5 8PP

Tel: 0115 967 2611   **Fax:** 0115 967 2642

Contact: David Williams

Health authority: Nottingham

Main business: To educate children aged 4–15 years on health issues

Life Education Centre Nottinghamshire

The centre is a mobile unit which visits 50 schools, based on a three-year spiral curriculum.

Contact: David Williams

Tel: 0115 967 2611

Partners: Rotary Club; Nottingham Health Authority; North Nottinghamshire Health Authority; North Nottinghamshire Tec; police; Local Education Authority

Funders: Local charities; North Nottinghamshire Tec

Target age group: 11–16

Target groups: Parents; neighbourhoods; community groups; rural communities

Methods and evaluation: Sessions are held in the mobile unit using hi-tech equipment – TV, video, laser disc, star ceiling, and work books.

Evaluation is by teachers, children, and educators.

NOTTINGHAM BDI (BLACK DRUG INITIATIVE)

4th Floor, Fenchurch House, 12 King Street, Nottingham NG1 2AS

Tel: 0115 941 0481   **Fax:** 0115 941 0481

Contact: Maria Ward

Health authority: Nottingham

Other drug services: Community safety; criminal justice; training; black prisoners' support

Main business: To provide projects in response to the needs of the black community

Peer education project

The project is based on the intake of 12 young people (14–25 years) from the Asian/Afro-Caribbean community who undertake peer education, personal development and drug awareness training (accredited course), and work as peer educators on completion.

Contact: Sharon Bowen

Tel: 0115 941 0481

Partners: Phoenix Project; Derby and Leicester Drug Action Team

Funders: East Midlands Drug Prevention Team; Crime Prevention

Target age groups: 14–25

Target groups: Offenders; black Caribbean; black African; black other; Indian; Pakistani; Bangladeshi; not at school; homeless; children in care

Methods and evaluation: The course includes modules on: personal development; street drug awareness, society, drugs and black communities; and peer education. Workshop settings use videos, discussion, role-play activities and the shared experiences of participants. The course is accredited by the Open College Network, and all participants must complete all areas and produce a portfolio of their work. Peer educators undertake a number of activities on completion, and may have an input into the next course.

The course will be researched by the Drug Prevention Initiative; and has been agreed at a national level to enable a comparison with other similar projects.

THE ZONE YOUTH PROJECT

St Martha's Vicarage, Frinton Road, Broxtowe, Nottingham NG8 6GR

Tel: 0115 927 8837

Contact: Roger Williams

Health authority: Nottingham

Net Café and street outreach work

Initiatives involve making contact with young people at risk in the 14–25 age band; working with small networking groups; creating alternative street activities; providing information; and providing a chemical-free café on Friday nights.

Contacts: Rob Burton, Israel Silgram

Tel: 0115 976 5138

Funders: Children In Need; National Lottery Charities Board

Needs assessment methods: A youth questionnaire in 1994 identified the top priority for young people as someone to listen to them, which led to the development of the café.

Target age groups: 14–25

Target groups: Offenders; users of heroin, cannabis; neighbourhoods

Evaluation: Evaluation is by a door-to-door/ street questionnaire.

Schools work and art events

These are initiatives to reach young people through schools, helping them to engage in life issues, including choices related to drugs and other damaging substances and lifestyles, and to use the arts to create a fresh focus for the area.

Contact: Rob Burton

Tel: 0115 976 5138

Partners: Local schools; youth and leisure services

Funder: National Lottery Charities Board

Needs assessment methods: A youth questionnaire in 1995 showed boredom amongst youths (leading to youth riots in 1993/4). These arts events aim to provide a fresh focus and network venues for outreach/street workers.

Target age groups: 11 and over

Target groups: Not at school; neighbourhoods

Methods and evaluation: Methods include putting on shows, activities and band nights, which utilise local talent and incorporate a wide variety of diversionary activities.

Evaluation is by questionnaire.

THE SAFE PROJECT (STREET ADVICE FOR EVERYONE)

Chandos Street, Netherfield, Nottinghamshire NG4 2LP

Tel: 0115 911 0338

Contact: Reverend Robin Old, Mel Dowson

Health authority: Nottingham

Other drug services: Community safety

Detached outreach work

The initiative involves working on the streets with young people, and befriending, supporting and advising them on any problems they have. It also offers education awareness around drug/alcohol misuse.

Contact: Mel Dowson, Shaun Holt

Tel: 0115 911 0338

Funders: East Midlands Drug Prevention Team; Nottingham City Council

Needs assessment methods: A need was identified from public consultation involving agencies, including police, Social Services, youth and community services and churches.

Target age groups: 11 and over

Target groups: Offenders; not at school; homeless; children in care; neighbourhoods; rural communities

Methods: Methods employed include: befriending and listening to young people; offering a free and confidential service; discussing drugs/drug-related issues with young people in an informal setting, concentrating on drug prevention and harm reduction; issuing leaflets on drug education/prevention to young people; and offering one-to-one support or counselling with young people.

The SAFE Project

The aim is to open an information and advice centre for young people.

Contacts: Mel Dowson, Shaun Holt

Tel: 0115 911 0338

Funders: Prince's Trust; Church of England Urban Fund

Needs assessment methods: there was a consultation between the Prince's Trust, church groups and committee members from SAFE.

Target age groups: 11 and over

Target groups: Not at school; homeless; neighbourhoods; rural communities.

Methods: An information and advice centre for young people will be opened offering a free and confidential service covering information, advice, support, counselling, and educational literature.

STUDENT SUPPORT GROUP

Hidcote, St James Manor, Long Bennington, Nottinghamshire NG23 5GZ

Tel: 01400 282507   **Fax:** 01400 282507

Contact: Shenagh Carling-Hay

Health authority: Lincolnshire

Student Support Group

The group aims: to educate young people about substance misuse; to raise awareness of substance misuse; to provide accurate and up-to-date information; to provide help and support.

Contact: Shenagh Carling-Hay

Tel: 01400 282507

Partners: Local secondary school

Funders: GADS (Grantham's Awareness of Drugs and Substances)

Target age groups: 11–18

Oxfordshire

ABINGDON DETACHED YOUTH WORK PROJECT

27 Bridge Street, Abingdon, Oxfordshire OX14 3HN

Tel: 01235 524755

Contact: Jon Ralph

Health authority: Oxfordshire

Drug education

The aim of this work is to provide young people with accurate and realistic information, and to support them in making informed choices.

Contact: Jon Ralph

Tel: 01235 524755

Partners: Schools; colleges; parents; police; District Council; nurses

Funders: Various; business sponsorship

Needs assessment methods: A lack of accurate information was identified. The 'Just say no' message was not relevant for those already using.

Target age groups: 11 and over

THAMES VALLEY POLICE, COMMUNITY AFFAIRS DEPARTMENT (BANBURY)

Police Station, Warwick Road, Banbury, Oxfordshire OX16 7AE

Tel: 01865 266697/8   **Fax:** 01865 266684

Contact: Police Constable Bob Goddard

Health authority: Oxfordshire

Other drug services: Community safety; criminal justice; training

Libra Project

This facility offers free and confidential information, support and counselling for people with problems arising from, or leading to, drugs or alcohol use.

Contact: Inspector Chris Mooney

Tel: 01865 266641

Partners: Banbury Crime Prevention Unit; Cherwell District Council; Oxfordshire Council on Alcohol and Drugs

Funders: Cherwell District Council; Banbury charities

YOUTH SERVICE

Community Education Office, The Mill, Spicebal Park, Banbury, Oxfordshire OX16 8QE

Tel: 01295 263942   **Fax:** 01295 263942

Contact: Judy Brown

Health authority: Oxfordshire

Other drug services: Training

The Bridge Information Project

The project aims to offer information and support to young people under 25 years. It has a major section on drugs education/information and aims to disseminate this to all youth projects in the area.

Contact: Kate Bird

Tel: 01295 272129

Funders: Oxfordshire County Council; Youth Service; donations from local businesses

Needs assessment methods: At an Oxfordshire conference, young people expressed the need for better access to information. A questionnaire was also sent out locally.

Target age groups: 11–25

Target group: Neighbourhoods

Methods: The information centre uses the National Youth Association System. Information is arranged around the walls of a coffee bar which is light, airy, and welcoming to young people. The shop is also the hub of the project and provides information (particularly on drugs) to other youth projects locally.

Missing Link – Theatre in Education (TIE) group

The group is involved in producing a play, to be toured to young people 14–19 years in schools/youth centres, accompanied by peer eduation workshops and a workshop pack for teachers/youth workers.

Contact: Polly Foster

Tel: 01295 252050

Partner: Mill Community Education Arts Centre

Funders: Mill Community Education Arts Centre; Cherwell District Council, Southern Arts, Prince's Trust

Needs assessment methods: All TIE members are users of the Mill. Discussion and debate with them around drugs issues resulted in this group.

Target age groups: 11–21

Target group: Parents

Methods: Several methods are employed, including: production of workshop materials in the form of a pack; encouragement of young people to form the TIE group and offer specific training; drugs awareness training for all participants via the Libra Project (drugs education project, p.192) – writing workshops with a community writer; producing a theatre piece with a writer; the writing of a drugs workshop pack for teachers, etc.; and the delivery of a play, touring and workshops.

Drugs were chosen as a topic because of relevance to theatre group and other young people.

THAMES VALLEY POLICE

Oxford Road, Kidlington, Oxfordshire OX5 2NX

Tel: 01865 846639   **Fax:** 01865 846630

Contact: David Purnell

Health authority: Oxfordshire

Other drug services: Community safety; criminal justice; training; arrest referral

Main business: Public safety; law and order; crime investigation and reduction

Oxfordshire Arrest Referral Scheme

This is a system that, at the point of arrest and detention, allows persons arrested for drug-related offences to be given details of an independent drug worker who will provide information about the services available to assist in behavioural change.

Contact: Phil Skillen

Tel: 01865 378999

Partners: Police; probation; Social Services; voluntary sector; Health Authority; Local Education Authority

Funders: Police Drug Action Team; Prince's Trust, Health Authority

Target groups: Offenders; white; black Caribbean; black African; black other; Indian; Pakistani; Bangladeshi; Chinese; other minority ethnic groups; homeless; children in care

Methods and evaluation: Young people are provided with a point of contact at a time of crisis. Working practices complement other agencies and good relationships for referral are being developed.

Evaluation is based on: the numbers taking up offers of help; the numbers not in treatment of other services; the numbers re-offering within 6–12 months. To date, 50 per cent of those contacting the scheme are not receiving any form of help.

AACYP (ASIAN AND AFRICAN CARIBBEAN YOUTH PROJECT)

Union Street Education Complex, Oxford OX4 1JP

Tel: 01865 251420

Contact: Ketan Gandhi

Health authority: Oxfordshire

Main business: Informal education for youth – life and social skills

Big Issue

This is an initiative to discuss aspects of the drug scene with young people, particularly in relation to dealing and using cannabis.

Contact: Ketan Gandhi

Tel: 01865 251420

Partners: Community Health Liaison Team; East Oxford Health Centre

Funders: Youth service; Health Authority

Target groups: Black Caribbean; black African; Indian; Pakistani; Bangladeshi; users of cannabis

Methods: The work on drugs is part of the broader work aimed at Asian young people who are at risk of criminality.

BOTLEY AREA YOUTH OFFICE

Matthew Arnold School, Cumnor, Oxford OX2 9JE

Tel: 01865 864717   **Fax:** 01865 864855

Contact: Jane Linthwaite

Health authority: Oxfordshire

Other drug services: Training on drug education and awareness for full-time and part-time workers

Rural Roadshow

The aim of the service is to provide young people with accurate, un-biased information on drugs through a participative session involving them in making choices on drug- and alcohol-related behaviour. It also aims to provide a service for young people in rural areas.

Contact: Jane Linthwaite

Tel: 01865 864717

Funders: Youth service; Thames Valley Partnership

Needs assessment methods: These took the form of questionnaires to young people, informal talks with young people, and feedback from part-time workers.

Target age groups: 11–21

Target group: Rural communities

Methods and evaluation: There are a variety of approaches, including: forum theatre techniques; discussions; quizzes; participative games; and creating written resources, leaflets and posters.

An evaluation report is written by the staff involved, based on questionnaires and verbal feedback from young people.

CAMPUS YOUTH CENTRE

The Primary School, Berinsfield, Oxford OX10 7LZ

Tel: 01863 340301   **Fax:** 01863 340301

Contact: Ken Chrisp

Health authority: Oxfordshire

Main business: Running a youth service provision for 9–25-year-olds

Campus Youth Centre

Hosts drug discussions for small groups of young people.

Contact: Ken Chrisp

Tel: 01863 340301

Partner: Health Authority

Funder: Health Authority

Needs assessment methods: A need was identified through listening to members and noting awareness of staff of a need to offer drug issues to members.

Target age groups: 9–25

Target groups: Neighbourhoods; rural communities

Methods: There are visits by professionals, who present a wide range of anti-drug measures. In addition, drama is used involving a professional youth worker who looks at a number of problems, and drugs is one of the main issues.

OCADU (OXFORDSHIRE COUNCIL ON ALCOHOL AND DRUG USE)

St Wres, Oxford Road, Cowley, Oxford OX4 2EN

Tel: 01865 749800   **Fax:** 01865 395250

Contact: Tony Woolman

Health authority: Oxfordshire

Other drug services: Treatment; criminal justice; training

Public campaign work

The aim of the work was: to inform communities about substance use and about services that offer information/support; to reduce harm for young people (under 25 years) using drugs; to provide publicly accessible information stalls/events. The project finished in March 1997.

Contact: Jason Mahoney

Tel: 01865 749800

Partners: Youth service; voluntary sector agencies; health/welfare workers at universities

Funders: Oxfordshire Health Authority; Oxfordshire Health Promotion Unit/Service

Target age groups: 11–25

Methods and evaluation: Information stalls (staffed) are presented in public areas where young people are able to easily access the information workers. Settings include street work, and venues such as youth clubs, shopping centres, and recreation/leisure venues. Information is provided about substances, risk reduction and services through posters, leaflets and discussion with workers.

Training and education

The aim was to offer training/education work about substance use to the communities of Oxfordshire, particularly young people, parents and professional groups, through experiential learning models and methods. The project finished in March 1997.

Contact: Jason Mahoney

Tel: 01865 749800

Funders: Schools and community groups

Methods and evaluation: Training is tailored according to the needs of the purchaser/ learners. Work with young people is primarily about learning to reduce risk, negotiating and seeking support. With parents, the focus is primarily about talking with a child and supporting young people in need. With professional groups/teams, the focus is usually about appropriate responses to drug use, but may be a more simple drugs awareness session where basic information is shared and attitudes are explored. All training uses experiential learning methods.

Evaluation questionnaires are administered to each group worked with to check the response to the workshop(s).

COMMUNITY EDUCATION SERVICE – VALE

King Alfred's Centre Site, Portway, Wantage, Oxfordshire OX12 GBY

Tel: 01235 762356   **Fax:** 01235 771009

Contact: Ruth Ashwell

Health authority: Oxfordshire

Other drug services: Community safety; training

Main business: Youth service – personal, social and political education across a whole range of issues and young people

Youth Information Strategy – survival guide

Part of a county-wide strategy for improving young people's access to information (including information on drugs), local projects include the publication of a survival guide and a phone information line.

Contact: Ruth Ashwell

Tel: 01235 762356

Funder: Youth service

Needs assessment methods: a questionnaire was sent to young people.

Target age groups: 11 and over

Methods: The strategy is a national co-ordination attempt. The two specific projects which provide information to all young people are: a survival guide (publication distributed to all school leavers in Oxfordshire, containing information on a range of issues); free phone information line offering confidential information and support to young people.

WANTAGE YOUTH CENTRE – THE SWEATBOX

King Alfred's School East, Springfield Road, Wantage, Oxfordshire OX12 8ES

Tel: 01235 763863

Contact: Garry Kingett

Health authority: Oxfordshire

Main business: Youth and community work

Drugs 'n' Pubs

The project aims to increase awareness in the Wantage area, and to provide appropriate information to young people in social environments where drug use is common.

Contact: Garry Kingett

Tel: 01235 763863

Funders: Oxford City Council Youth Services; Vale of White Horse District Council Health Advisory Group

Needs assessment methods:
Questionnaires and direct contact and discussion with young people in pubs and clubs showed a perceived increase in availability and use of drugs by young people; as well as a lack of knowledge and awareness over various aspects of drug use.

Target age groups: 11 and over

Target groups: Offenders; neighbourhoods; rural communities

Methods: Youth workers contacted and discussed drugs education with young people in seven local pubs and clubs. Supporting educational material (Lifeline) was introduced, and evaluated by young people. Arrangements were made with landlords/managers to have permanent drugs information and advice racks installed in pubs. The information includes local county and national contact points.

THE FLAT: COUNSELLING AND INFORMATION SERVICE

Old Police Station, Church Green, Witney, Oxfordshire OX8 6AW

Tel: 01993 702060

Contacts: Debbie Lee, Nick Luxmoore

Health authority: Oxfordshire

Other drug services: Treatment; training

Main business: Counselling and information

Counselling and information

The service aims to provide accurate information and high-quality counselling to young people.

Contacts: Debbie Lee, Nick Luxmoore

Tel: 01993 702060

Funders: Oxfordshire County Council; local health service, charities; agencies.

Needs assessment methods: A pilot project was undertaken as well as a conference of all major agencies.

Methods and evaluation: Methods include drop-in sessions and pre-arranged counselling appointments.

Evaluation is by record forms which are completed for each contact and analysed. There is also a questionnaire sent to all major local agencies.

Somerset

OFF THE RECORD (BATH)

Open House Centre, Manvers Street, Bath, Somerset BA1 1VW

Tel: 01225 312481   **Fax:** 01225 312481

Contact: Clare Chapman

Health authority: Avon

Other drug services: Treatment; short- and long-term person-centred counselling/therapy work

Main business: General information, advice and counselling service for young people aged 13–25

Group work activities

The object is to provide a safe place to explore attitudes, knowledge and behaviour, in relation to drugs, through group discussion, questionnaires, games, etc. It aims to raise awareness in terms of preventing drug use from starting, to inform, to minimise harm and to support efforts at stopping. Funding for the activity ceased at the end of March 1996.

Contact: Clare Chapman

Tel: 01225 312481

Funder: Young People at Risk from Drugs (DoH grant scheme)

Needs assessment methods: A questionnaire was sent to approximately 120 young people in order to ascertain if they would visit the Drugs Information Resources Room and what resources/information they would like to see.

Target age groups: 13–25

Target groups: Parents and professionals, e.g. teachers

Methods and evaluation: Group work

activities involve discussion, quizzes, card games, videos, board games, information search, and case studies. Two workers lead the session by involving the participants and seeking their views, attitudes and knowledge of drugs. Participants' responses are monitored through an anonymous questionnaire, which provides evidence of increased awareness and knowledge of (or lack of) drugs, and any change in attitude and behaviour in terms of starting, reducing or stopping drug use.

Evaluation was carried out by training organisations involved with activity, i.e. Bath Area Drugs Advisory Service and NACRO South West as well as by participants and staff.

It involves: a questionnaire completed by all participants or by verbal responses; evaluation reports provided by training organisations indicating changes in skills, knowledge and behaviour with clients; and an independent evaluation report and summary report of statistical returns made by the Innovation Group.

STRATAGEM – CONSULTANCY AND TRAINING FOR SENSITIVE ISSUES

161 Englishcombe Lane, Bath, Somerset BA2 2EL

Tel: 01380 733822   **Fax:** 01380 733760

Contact: Shelagh Hetreed

Health authority: Avon

The Bath Young People's Peer-Led Research Project

The aims of the project were to equip a group of young people with the skills to: conduct research among their peer groups on gender differences in drug behaviour; consider their findings, select the most important issues and design a one-day conference for other young people; learn how to facilitate small groups through structured exercises. The project finished in May 1996.

Contact: Shelagh Hetreed

Tel: 01380 733822

Funders: Bath and Wiltshire Health Commission; Social Services; Bath City Council and Avon Constabulary

Needs assessment methods: A meeting of the Bath Alliance prioritised action plans – work involving young people was one priority.

Target age groups: 11–21

Target group: Teachers

Methods and evaluation: 20 young researchers worked in three settings (two single-sex schools and one youth and community centre). They met weekly for two months and: designed and used their own research questionnaires to establish perceived drug-related behaviour in peer groups; used collected data to identify key issues for a conference; decided on suitable strategies for promoting discussion (e.g. card sorting, stand point talking); created suitable exercises; established a programme for the day; and learned how to lead small groups. The conference had an attendance of 130 young people and was peer led. Issues for individual groups were written on transparencies and presented by each group at the final plenary.

All participants completed an evaluation through written questionnaires and interviews at the end of the conference. A sample of the group leaders plus participants will be interviewed to assess the impact on their lives/schools in the medium term.

SCAT (SOMERSET COLLEGE OF ARTS AND TECHNOLOGY)

Wellington Road, Taunton, Somerset TA1 5AX

Tel: 01823 366366   **Fax:** 01823 366418

Contact: Virginia Eccles

Health authority: Somerset

Other drug services: Training

Main business: Higher Education and Further Education College

SCAT's drug information project

A project under which students from courses throughout the college produce and market a range of drug education material directed to other students and young people. The project finished in June 1997.

Contact: Virginia Eccles

Tel: 01823 366366

Funder: Bristol Drug Prevention Team

Needs assessment methods: A questionnaire survey targeted 500 students, selected at random across the college.

Target age groups: 11 and over

SOMERSET COUNTY YOUTH SERVICE

Training and Development, Weir Lodge, 83 Staplegrove Road, Taunton, Somerset TA1 1DN

Tel: 01823 252089   **Fax:** 01823 332678

Contact: Glenda Adamson/Helge Maul

Health authority: Somerset

Other drug services: Training

Peer education (drugs prevention)

These initiatives deal with groups of young people in the 15–20-year age range, supporting them in devising, developing and delivering drugs messages to their peers through a variety of media.

Contact: Glenda Adamson

Tel: 01823 252089

Funders: Grants for Education Support and Training funding; Somerset County Council, town and district councils; Drug Prevention Initiative

Needs assessment methods: A research project: found the level of drug use amongst young people in Somerset in the 15–20-year age range.

Target age groups: 15–20

Methods and evaluation: Part-time workers are recruited to support local groups, which are trained and supported through centrally co-ordinated residential and one-day events. These events take young people through social education process based on a high participation with drugs and focus on the effect, the legal and health implications. Young people choose from a variety of media, develop projects (allocation of development money), and agree to deliver to a minimum of three peer groups.

Evaluation is by participants of delivery sessions, as well as pre- and post-course questionnaires/ worker reviews.

THE GENESIS YOUTH THEATRE GROUP

The Arts Centre, Eight Acre Lane, Wellington, Somerset TA21 8PS

Tel: 01823 667701

Contact: Colin Frost

Health authority: Somerset

Main business: Theatre

The Genesis Youth Theatre Group

The aim is to develop theatre skills for peer education.

Contact: Colin Frost

Tel: 01823 666548

Funders: Home Office Drug Prevention Initiative; Wellington Arts Association

Target age groups: 11–18

Target groups: Parents (in particular Arts Association parents); schools

Methods: Methods include: drug training and peer education; training in theatre skills; community and parental awareness; talks; and workshops.

WEST SOMERSET PARENTS AND RURAL COMMUNITIES PROJECT

49 Howard Road, Wellington, Somerset TA21 8RX

Tel: 01823 666548   **Fax:** 01823 666548

Contact: Colin Frost

Health authority: Somerset

Other drug services: Treatment; criminal justice; training

SPARC

The project aims to inform and assist the parents and rural community of West Somerset in all areas of drug misuse, information and support, and to raise the awareness of the community as a whole.

Contact: Colin Frost

Tel: 01823 666548

Funders: Home Office Drug Prevention Initiative; apa

Needs assessment methods: A Home Office survey found concerns over parental knowledge about drugs.

Target groups: Parents; neighbourhoods; community groups; rural communities

Methods and evaluation: Methods include leaflet distribution, talks, displays, and training of other workers; education and training of parents to run support groups; telephone and caller support – limited to areas of most need; interactive sessions for parents at meeting rooms in communities; the promotion of community development by actively engaging in groups; support and training sessions for professionals.

Ongoing surveys with professionals, business community, parents and contacts continually evaluate the project.

SAFE HOUSE

c/o Turning Point, 1–5 Broad Street, Wells, Somerset BA5 2DJ

Tel: 01749 677791   **Fax:** 01749 679109

Contact: Nick Ross

Health authority: Somerset

Safe House

The project aims to provide information, advice and support in clubs and at private parties for people involved in dance culture, as well as alternative therapies, water, condoms, etc., and to ensure adequate provision of water, ventilation, heating control, and safety in clubs.

Contact: Nick Ross

Tel: 01749 677791

Partners: Turning Point; Somerset AIDS Advice; County Youth Service; DANCE

Funders: Drug Action Team; Drug Prevention Team (Somerset), Community chest

Needs assessment methods: the need for this project arose out of going to clubs, circulating questionnaires, and talking to club goers, promoters and managers about the service needs and the current service provisions. Other groups involved in work at raves were also contacted.

Target age groups: 17 and over

Target groups: Users of amphetamines, dance drugs; ravers, promoters, managers

Methods: The project provides the following: a 'chill out' environment in clubs and at private parties, incorporating a stall/displays and information leaflets, articles, etc., about drug use and related issues; alternative therapies – shiatsu, aromatherapy, reflexology; free fruit and condoms, comfortable seating, i.e. creating a safe space; face-to-face support/information available at information stalls and around club/party; staff to check heating/ventilation, water availability, if anyone is feeling unwell, and to offer first aid; and support/advice for promoters/managers to make venues as safe as possible.

YOUNG SOMERSET

Old School, Westonwycand, Somerset TA7 0LN

Tel: 01278 691999   **Fax:** 01278 691912

Contact: Ian Wallace

Health authority: Somerset

Other drug services: Training; information to young people

Main business: Youth work

Peer education programme

The programme aims to work with a group of young people so that they can be pro-active in developing and delivering a health education programme to other young people.

Contact: Ian Wallace

Tel: 01278 691999

Partner: Somerset Youth Service

Funders: Drug Prevention Team; District Council

Target age groups: 11–18

Target groups: Community groups (in particular two towns in Somerset)

Methods: A core group is preparing two youth health days at which agencies will have a stall, and the county drugs prevention peer education groups will present workshops, drama and videos, and provide an alcohol-free bar and a disco/social event.

Staffordshire

PRIDE (PEOPLE REDUCING THE INFLUENCE OF DRUGS BY EDUCATION)

F Dept, Community Service, Police HQ, Cannock Road, Stafford ST17 0QG

Tel: 01785 232535   **Fax:** 01785 232369

Contact: Police Constable Nigel Jackson

Health authority: Staffordshire

Other drug services: Community safety; criminal justice; training

PRIDE (Working Together in Partnership)

The initiative is to reduce the influence of drugs by education.

Contact: Police Constable Nigel Jackson

Tel: 01785 232535

Funder: Self-funding

Target group: Multi-agency partnership

DRUGLINK NORTH STAFFORDSHIRE

76-82 Hope St, Hanley, Stoke-on-Trent, Staffordshire ST1 5BX

Tel: 01782 202139   **Fax:** 01782 201553

Contact: Tom Jackson

Health authority: North Staffordshire

Other drug services: Treatment; criminal justice; training; needle exchange; advocacy; young persons' clinic; aromatherapy

Cobridge Single Regeneration Project

The project aims to develop services for a specific area under Stoke Borough Council in conjunction with a range of specifically funded projects.

Contact: Tom Jackson

Tel: 01782 202139

Partner: Housing Association

Funder: Single Regeneration Budget

Needs assessment methods: Interviews were conducted with drug users in outreach settings.

Target age groups: 11 and over

Target groups: Black Caribbean; black African; black other; Indian; Pakistani; Bangladeshi; neighbourhoods

Methods and evaluation: The primary focus is on contacting clients in outreach settings – on streets, in parks, in clubs and at other venues. The work is face-to-face, with the additional provision of condoms, needle exchange and a leaflet. Peer education is currently being developed.

Evaluation is to be established following research results.

Mobile service

The aim of the mobile service, which covers a wide geographical area, is: to make the Druglink service more accessible; to demystify/promote the Druglink service; to contact drug-users not already in contact with a service; to provide advice/information on drug-related issues and HIV infection; and to provide needle exchange in appropriate venues.

Contacts: Paula Hammond, Tom Jackson

Tel: 01782 202139

Partner: Staffordshire Probation Service

Funders: HIV and Sexual Health Unit; Staffordshire Probation Service

Needs assessment methods: Before the mobile service goes into an area, the following are considered: what services are already available in the area?; the distance from a Druglink centre; any recent media publicity; requests from residents and clients already using the service.

Target age groups: 17 and over

Target groups: Offenders; when parked outside probation offices, the service is still open to the general public.

Evaluation: Evaluation is by: questionnaires completed by independent researchers; monthly statistics; and the Home Office, via interviews of staff and clients.

Outreach work

Outreach involves making contact with young people not otherwise in touch with the centre in order to provide information and practical support on drugs/drug use, HIV and other sexually transmitted diseases.

Contacts: Tom Jackson, Steve Morrey

Tel: 01782 202139

Funders: HIV and sexual health units

Needs assessment methods: When an area or venue is being considered for outreach, reports in the media and centre-based referrals information from clients help to build a picture of the suitability of the work.

Target age groups: 17 and over

Evaluation: Independent research questionnaires; database statistics; independent research; and Home Office interviews are all used.

Women's project

The project targets its work on women, including those working in the sex industry.

Contact: Jacquie Johnson, Tom Jackson

Tel: 01782 202139

Partners: Health Authority; HIV/Sexual Health Promotion Unit/Service

Funders: Health Authority; Single Regeneration Budget

Needs assessment methods: An assessment carried out by the Health Authority highlighted a strong association between women working on the streets and drug use.

Target groups: Women; neighbourhoods

Methods: There is outreach in locations where women are known to work, involving face-to-face contact, and condom and needle/syringe provision. There is also a regular drop-in clinic at the current women's centre in the city.

Suffolk

ST EDMUNDSBURY SUBSTANCE MISUSE GROUP

Borough Offices, Angel Hill, Bury St Edmunds, Suffolk IP33 1XB

Tel: 01284 757233   **Fax:** 01284 757124

Contact: D Rendle

Health authority: Suffolk

Other drug services: Training; information provision; consciousness training; community strategy

Main business: Alcohol and tobacco

Drug Education Week

The activities aimed to raise awareness of drug misuse, focusing on parents. The week included: displays in all major venues in the town; radio interviews with members of the planning group; and a video project sponsored by Anglia TV at King Edward VI School. The outcome was used to publicise a major activity week in July 1997.

Contact: Ian Miles

Tel: 01284 761393

Partners: St Edmundsbury Borough Council; community education; Mid Anglia NHS Trust; middle and upper schools in West Sussex

Funders: Tesco, Marks & Spencer; St Edmundsbury Borough Council

Target age group: 11–16

Target group: Parents

Methods: The activities included: project work for display in schools and drama presentations; beer mats, posters and provision of leaflets; video productions and a video competition for 1997; interviews and a discussion on local radio; and a disco for drugs awareness.

MID-SUFFOLK DISTRICT COUNCIL

131 High Street, Needham Market, Ipswich, Suffolk IP6 8DL

Tel: 01449 720711   **Fax:** 01449 727237

Contact: Christine Jackson

Health authority: Suffolk

Stowmarket Drugs Forum

The forum is an inter-agency approach to tackling drug misuse.

Contact: Dr Tony Froud

Tel: 01449 613541

Partners: Police; churches; town and district councils; Drugs Advisory Service; Health Authority; air base; youth service; Local Education Authority; Health Authority

Funders: Police; local authority; Drugs Advisory Service; Health Authority; air base; youth service; Local Education Authority

Target groups: Parents; neighbourhoods; community groups; rural communities

Methods: The forum held a drug awareness week, which involved a mobile exhibition centre staffed by participating organisations, together with parents'/open evenings at the local schools.

Walsham Le Willows – pilot project

This is a community initiative.

Contact: Christine Jackson

Tel: 01449 720711

Partners: Parish council; drug squad; GP practice; Drugs Advisory Service; Schools; Parent–Teachers Association; local authority

Funder: Local authority

Needs assessment methods: Methods used were: a literature search; contact with relevant agencies; and questionnaires to all inhabitants.

Target groups: Parents; neighbourhoods; community groups; rural communities

Methods and evaluation: The project employs the following: public meetings; questionnaires; parents' meetings; and publicity.

Evaluation is by questionnaire.

SUFFOLK COMMUNITY ALCOHOL SERVICES (SCAS)

41 Lower Brook Street, Ipswich, Suffolk IP4 1AQ

Tel: 01473 259382   **Fax:** 01473 289471

Contact: M Jeffries

Health authority: Suffolk

Other drug services: Criminal justice; focus of agency is alcohol misuse, but in terms of educational work it falls within the sphere of substance misuse

Suffolk Probation Service Partnership

Under the partnership, Suffolk Community Alcohol Services (SCAS) provides an input to the Suffolk Probation Service (SPS). A groupwork programme has developed.

Contact: R Forrest

Tel: 01473 259382

Partner: Suffolk Probation Service

Funder: Suffolk Probation Service

Needs assessment methods: Needs assessment within the Suffolk Probation Service has been developed over time by Carey Godfrey. There was 8 per cent recidivism after a year.

Target group: Offenders

Methods and evaluation: The groupwork programme was originally submitted to the Home Office by SCAS, and was subsequently modified by Suffolk Probation Service. It is a series of ten sessions focusing on a variety of aspects of substance misuse.

The outcome of this work has been evaluated by SCAS up to April 1996, when Suffolk Probation Service took up this responsibility. Reports to Suffolk Probation Service on this were regularly provided. Evaluation has been through knowledge questionnaires and the occurrence of recidivism.

Young People and Substance Misuse Project

The project focuses on young people known to the social services department and probation as being at risk of harm through substance misuse.

Contact: M Jeffries

Tel: 01473 259382

Partners: Social Services department; probation

Funder: Department of Health

Target age groups: 11 and over

Target group: Those known to the Social Services department/probation

Methods and evaluation: Methods include: motivational work; alternatives to drug use; and group discussion.

Evaluation is through meetings between funder/managing body/Social Services department/probation managers, and takes the form of a pre-arranged knowledge questionnaire on a readiness to change.

SUFFOLK COUNTY COUNCIL – COMMUNITY EDUCATION

Education Department, St Andrew House, County Hall, Ipswich, Suffolk IP4 1LJ

Tel: 01473 264610   **Fax:** 01473 264610

Contact: Steve Oldacre

Health authority: Suffolk

Main business: Community education including youth work, adult education and community development

Detached youth work project

This project aims to work with young people on the streets and any other places where they congregate in Newmarket.

Contact: Suzanne Pearson

Tel: 01638 663740

Partner: Forest Heath District Council

Funders: Forest Heath District Council; Suffolk County Council

Needs assessment methods: A pilot project was set up after initial interest was aroused from a report identifying needs.

Target age groups: 11 and over

Target groups: Homeless; neighbourhoods; rural communities

Methods and evaluation: First the project tries to gain the trust of young people who have no meeting base, and then use informal discussions, questionnaires and games to challenge and expand the knowledge of the young people.

Evaluation is by participants, staff and Richard Spring, MP, and takes the form of discussions with all participants; practical observation; record keeping; monthly staff meetings/debriefs.

Saxmundham Drugs Project

The project involved working with young people aged 14–18 years to research drug issues and to design preventative material for 11–14-year-olds. It ran until March 1996.

Contact: Helen Muddoch

Tel: 01728 602689

Funder: Local Education Authority

Needs assessment methods: A need for the project arose out of face-to-face work with young people.

Target age groups: 11–18

Target groups: Users of dance drugs; not at school; rural communities

Methods and evaluation: A group of young people gathered over several weeks to evaluate current information/leaflets which dealt with drugs misuse. They then suggested better ways to get the message across to younger people – such as posters, clothing, stickers, cards, etc. The group then set about devising such information, thereby learning about drugs and the consequence of their misuse.

The end product was actually used to evaluate the process. Results and impact on individuals are hard to measure.

Young Men's Health Promotion Roadshow

The aim is to increase the reliable information current amongst young men in the 14–20 age bracket, so as to promote healthy choices, through visiting youth groups in the North Suffolk education area.

Contact: Les Cockrill

Tel: 01728 832477

Partners: Health Promotion Development Fund; Suffolk Health Authority; East Suffolk MIND; Community Drugs Team; Suffolk Association of Youth

Funders: Health Promotion Development Fund; community education; Health Promotion and Education

Needs assessment methods: A need arose from extractions from existing studies in relation to men's health promotion and rural access to information. Others involved with similar work were also consulted.

Target age groups: 14–20

Target groups: Males; rural communities

Evaluation: Evaluation is through a questionnaire for participants; nightly recordings by project staff; and reports from those units visited.

Young Persons' Health Education Workers' Project

The project aims to promote health and healthy lifestyles among young people through education, empowerment and encouragement. Health workers present informal education in youth club settings.

Contact: Patsy Little

Tel: 01502 538038

Partners: Health Promotion Unit/Service; community education

Funders: Health Authority (through James Paget Trust); Suffolk Community Education

Needs assessment methods: Surveys, consultation and statistics revealed the need for access to accurate health information on a variety of health issues, as well as for better knowledge of the services available.

Target age groups: 11–21

Target group: Homeless

Methods and evaluation: Methods used include: video and discussion; discussion groups; visits to appropriate agencies; board games; drama; short courses; one-to-one discussion; and posters and artwork.

The project is evaluated via a health adviser, including analysis of sessional records, a survey of the young people involved, and a survey of the youth-worker line managers.

SUFFOLK PROBATION SERVICE

Foundation House, 34 Foundation Street, Ipswich, Suffolk IP4 1SP

Tel: 01473 210675   **Fax:** 01473 236212

Contact: Carey Godfrey

Health authority: Suffolk

Other drug services: Criminal justice; training

Main business: Preparing reports for courts and supervising young offenders

Alcohol and Drug Education Awareness Group

The group aims: to increase knowledge and awareness of the consequences of using and misusing alcohol and drugs; to reduce the risk of self-harm; and to reduce offending levels.

Contact: Carey Godfrey

Tel: 01473 210675

Partner: Suffolk Community Alcohol Services

Funder: Suffolk Probation Service

Needs assessment methods: The assessment was based on probation clients with a substance misuse problem.

Target group: Offenders

Methods and evaluation: The group bases its work on groupwork with a ten-week course facililated by Suffolk Probation Service and Suffolk Community Alcohol Services. The course has two-hour sessions, involving information giving, exercises, videos, and motivational interviewing.

Evaluation is through the following: the number of referrals; attendance; objective measure of level of knowledge; readiness to change indicators; group members' evaluation, probation officers' evaluation; and re-offending levels.

STOWMARKET DRUGS FORUM

Church Road, Stowupland, Stowmarket, Suffolk IP30 9TU

Tel: 01449 242553 **Fax:** 01449 774859 **e-mail:** stowupld@mailboxrmplc.co.uk

Contact: C Whyatt

Health authority: Suffolk

Drugs awareness-raising week for parents

The week aimed to provide parents with the necessary information and skills to enable them to talk about drugs with their children. This project ran in June 1996.

Contact: C Whyatt

Tel: 01449 242553

Partners: Health Authority; Community Drugs Team; Army Welfare; Local Education Authority; County Council; ADFAM; other charitable groups

Funders: Voluntary contributions

Target groups: Parents; neighbourhoods; rural communities

Methods and evaluation: Several activities during the week included: leaflets to parents; a sponsored cash prize for the drugs quiz; presentations from the police/Community Drugs Team; group sessions for parents; and counselling sessions, if required. There was also a touring caravan.

An evaluation sheet, devised by Suffolk Health authority, was sent to all parents attending evening sessions.

ADFAM (SUFFOLK)

PO Box 35, Woodbridge, Suffolk IP12 4NW

Tel: 01394 460001

Contact: Christina Oakley

Health authority: Suffolk

Other drug services: Training; support services for anyone affected by drug misuse, particularly parents, families, partners, etc.

Peer and preventative education

The education activities aim: to raise awareness of the effects drug misuse has on the families and friends of the misuser; to inform young people of the dangers of drug misuse for physical and mental health; and to encourage people to take responsibility for their decisions and actions, past and present.

Contacts: Tony Booth/Lilias Sheershanks

Tel: 01394 460001

Partners: Community Education; police; Community Safety Team/Unit; probation and prison service

Funders: Health Authority; Social Services, charitable trusts, schools

Needs assessment methods: Contact with school liaison officers, and meetings with statutory and voluntary agencies from East Anglia established that there was no agency involved with the needs of young people and their families.

Target age groups: 11 and over

Target groups: Offenders; not at school; homeless; children in care; parents; neighbourhoods; community groups (urban and rural)

Methods and evaluation: The activities use the following methods: using peer educators with 'hands-on' experience to conduct workshops in a group setting in schools/youth clubs/young offenders' institutions, etc.; using schools liaison officers in three main areas of Suffolk to act as contacts for schools in those areas; providing individual pupils, or other young people identified as needing support with drug/substance problem, with an experienced support worker for a specified period (in agreement with school/parents); acting as an independent mediator between school/pupil/parents (parents must be agreeable).

Evaluation is by verbal and written feedback from pupils and teachers in schools, and from health co-ordinators in young offenders' institutions.

Surrey

MAYFLOWER OUTREACH PROJECT

Frith Cottage, Church Road, Frimley, Surrey GU16 5AD

Tel: 01276 670883   **Fax:** 01276 679474

Contact: Anne M Bell

Health authority: West Surrey

Other drug services: Treatment; needle exchanges, steroids focus

Pubs and clubs work

The basis of this work is providing information and advice sessions on drugs and HIV, including sessions at clubs, to prevent problematic drug use.

Contact: Anne M Bell

Tel: 01276 670883

Partners: Surrey Youth Service; Surrey Police

Funders: Acorn; Surrey Youth Service

Target group: Users of dance drugs

Methods: Methods involved include: attendance at dance venues throughout the authority area; information and advice on recreational drug use; harm minimisation leaflets and condom distribution; and the opportunity to talk to two outreach workers on drug use.

SURREY POLICE

Surrey Police HQ, Mount Browne, Sandy Lane, Guildford, Surrey GU3 1HG

Tel: 01483 571212   **Fax:** 01483 300279

Contact: Peter Nightingale

Health authority: West Surrey

Other drug services: Community safety; criminal justice; training

Main business: Law enforcement; order maintenance; community safety

MANDATE (Multi-Agency Drugs and Alcohol Training and Education)

The project aims to provide education and training in relation to the misuse of drugs and alcohol.

Contact: Peter Nightingale

Tel: 01483 482759

Funders: MANDATE agencies; Safer Surrey Partnership

Needs assessment methods: An assessment of the provision involved gap analysis, and a feasibility study, and resulted in the need for a co-ordinated philosophy and approach.

Target age groups: 11 and over

Target group: Parents

ROYAL BOROUGH OF KINGSTON-UPON-THAMES

The Guildhall, Kingston-upon-Thames, Surrey KT1 1EU

Tel: 0181 547 6099   **Fax:** 0181 547 6004

Contact: Grahame Snelling

Health authority: Kingston and Richmond

Other drug services: Treatment; community safety; criminal justice; training

Main business: Providing services for children in need and those who need to be looked after

Young people at risk from drugs

Jointly run with the local community NHS trust, this project aimed to work with targeted groups of young people whose drug use was becoming problematic, and for whom a harm minimisation programme was appropriate. It also provided information sessions for carers to minimise placement breakdown. The project finished in May 1996.

Contact: Grahame Snelling

Tel: 0181 547 6099

Partners: Kingston and District NHS Community Trust

Funders: Young People at Risk from Drugs

(Department of Health's grant scheme); Health Authority, Kingston children's services

Needs assessment methods:
Questionnaires were sent to case-holding social workers of young people aged 12–18 years to determine problematic drug use. About 80 forms were sent out and returned. Some 30 young people in the target group were identified as having a problem with drug use as against a set of psychological testing indicators.

Target age groups: 12–18

Target groups: Children in care; parents and foster carers

YAP (YOUTH AWARENESS PROGRAMME) – MITCHAM

226 London Road, Mitcham, Surrey CR4 3HD

Tel: 0181 640 9736

Contact: Lee Harper-Penman

Health authority: Merton, Sutton and Wandsworth

Other drug services: Treatment; community safety; criminal justice; training; crime prevention

Graffiti Project

The aim is: to create an informal setting where young people may express their artistic talents; to provide drugs education and awareness within the workshops; and to offer counselling, support and advice to young people if needed.

Contact: Lee Harper-Penman

Tel: 0181 640 9736

Funders: Behavioural units, youth clubs

Target age groups: 11 and over

Target groups: Offenders; black Caribbean; black African; Indian; Pakistani; Bangladeshi; Chinese; users of amphetamines, crack/cocaine, cannabis; not at school; homeless; children in care; neighbourhoods; community groups (Merton Tenant Association); rural communities

Methods and evaluation: Evaluation is through forms.

Photographic project

The project aims to create an informal environment where young people can express their individuality, opinions and concerns, as well as develop their self-esteem and respect through their artistic talents, while at the same time accessing drugs education.

Contact: Lee Harper-Penman

Tel: 0181 640 9736

Funders: Youth clubs

Target group: Offenders

SUTTON YAP (YOUTH AWARENESS PROGRAMME)

103 Westmead Road, Sutton, Surrey SM1 4JD

Tel: 0181 770 0017   **Fax:** 0181 770 0211

Contact: Steven Baird

Health authority: Merton, Sutton and Wandsworth

Other drug services: Criminal justice; training; drug awareness and addiction training

Main business: Youth advice and information agency; also involved in setting up drug education programmes for parents

Drop-in centre/shop

The centre aims to contact young people in a non-intrusive manner, giving them information and advice on matters surrounding drugs and drug use, and to make them aware of YAP and the training and counselling available.

Contact: Ceri Hughes

Tel: 0181 770 0017

Funder: Sutton YAP

Target age groups: 11 and over

Target groups: Not at school; parents

Methods and evaluation: The shop is a first point of contact for many people, drug using and non-drug using adults and young people, and primarily provides written and verbal advice and information. It is also used as a point to redirect people back to the project for counselling, training or further information. People drop in, and cards are handed out around the centre to publicise the shop.

The St Nicholas Centre needed the unit back for 3 months, during which time it was considered how to make the shop appeal to young people.

Evaluation is through trying to find ways to improve contact by supplying more information about facilities for young people in the area, by talking with young people, and asking them what they wanted.

Drug awareness workshops

The workshops aim to provide confidential drug awareness and harm reduction advice to young people through venues such as schools, colleges, universities and youth provisions.

Contact: Steven Baird

Tel: 0181 770 0017

Funder: Sutton Borough Council

Needs assessment methods: Research was conducted through questionnaires and interviews amongst young people in the YAP area about what they wanted and needed from a drugs agency and where they got drugs information.

Target age groups: 11 and over

Methods and evaluation: Three workshops are carried out with young people looking at the psychological, economic, physiological and social effects, and the consequences of drug use. They allow the young people to ask questions around drugs and related issues in a safe, non-judgemental environment which provides them with harm minimisation information while dispelling any myths and misconceptions.

Recordings are made by the workshop leaders and the young people fill out evaluation forms. A separate evaluation is conducted by the Home Office.

Outreach work

The aim of this work is to meet young people on their own territories, informing them of the services available and providing them with confidential advice and information around drugs and related issues.

Contact: Marc Sayce

Tel: 0181 770 0017

Funder: Sutton Single Regeneration Budget

Needs assessment methods: An appraisal interview was carried out to assess primary activities and purposes, justification of need and monitoring arrangements.

Target age groups: 11 and over

Target group: Neighbourhoods

Methods and evaluation: The purpose of the work is to respond to young people on their own territories (on the street, arcades, etc.), providing them with confidential information and support around drugs and related issues. The work carried out focuses on the identified needs of young people, and involves liaising with different individuals and organisations within the local area. Workers also encourage young people to use the other services the agency offers.

Meetings are held with the funders, and financial monitoring and output forms are completed quarterly. An outreach evaluation form is completed after each session, which includes the number of young people contacted, their ethnic origin and the issues discussed.

Rave work

Initiatives involve working within raves and dance clubs to provide basic first-aid, harm reduction advice and 'talk down' service.

Contacts: Melanie Gray, Nicky Rollings

Tel: 0181 770 0017

Funders: Sutton YAP; London Borough of Sutton; Solotec; Single Regeneration Budget; South-west London Probation Service.

Target groups: Users of dance drugs; club goers

Methods: Volunteers are on hand at venues to provide immediate first-aid to clubbers until a qualified paramedic is available. Informal harm reduction advice and drug information is provided to those who seek it, and (depending on the specific contract with the club owners/ promoters) free water is provided to those who need it. Publicity materials, specifically designed to appeal to club goers, are also given out.

East Sussex

EAST SUSSEX EDUCATION AUTHORITY – PSE ADVISORY TEAM

Education Office, Royal York Building, The Old Steine, Brighton, East Sussex BN1 62A

Tel: 01273 820 150   **Fax:** 01273 736744

Contact: Ruth Hilton/Gillian Cunliffe

Health authority: East Sussex, Brighton and Hove

Other drug services: Training; inspection

Main business: Personal and social education

After-School RAP Club

The club provides vulnerable 'at risk' young people with diversionary activities and raises self-esteem.

Contact: Mandy Foyster

Tel: 01273 820150

Partners: East Sussex Drug Prevention Team; schools; youth service; Local Education Authority

Funders: Local Education Authority; Department for Education and Employment

Needs assessment methods: Interviews with school staff, were carried out.

Target age group: 11–16

Methods and evaluation: Vulnerable youngsters, at risk of drug abuse, are identified by school staff and then invited to attend an after-school club one day per week. Run by an experienced youth worker, the club seeks to raise the self-esteem and self-awareness of the young people through group work and diversionary activities.

The initiative is independently evaluated.

Peer education in two community colleges

The aims are: to establish a pilot peer-led drug programme within Year 12 to enable peer trainers to identify their own needs and those of their peer group; to train peer trainers; and to deliver peer education.

Contact: Gillian Cunliffe

Tel: 01273 820150

Partners: Health Promotion Unit/Service; Drug Prevention Team; school; youth service and advisory team

Funders: Drug Prevention Team; Local Education Authority

Needs assessment methods: A feasibility study was carried out by the project worker.

Target age groups: 11–21

Target group: Rural communities

Methods: The project involves training of the peer educators through a residential in-house induction week, and ongoing training and monitoring of the peer educators.

Power to the Parent course

The course is made up of six evening sessions for the parents/carers of young people, with the main aim of providing support and information for parents which will in turn be of benefit to young people.

Contact: Mandy Foyster

Tel: 01273 820150

Partners: East Sussex Drug Prevention Initative; Consortium

Funders: Local Education Authority; Department for Education and Employment

Needs assessment methods: Informal interviews were held with school staff as well as workshops with parents.

Target age group: 11–16

Evaluation: An independent evaluator used observational techniques, interviews and questionnaires.

PHASE

Premier House, 11 Marlborough Place, Brighton, East Sussex BN1 1UB

Tel: 01273 694040   **Fax:** 01903 716718

Contact: Raymond Burns

Health authority: East Sussex, Brighton and Hove

Other drug services: Treatment; community safety; criminal justice; parent work

Main business: Drugs and alcohol – information, advice, support and outreach

Parent Drug Advice Network (PDAN)

The network aims to: provide information, support and advice to parents about drugs and their children; educate parents through drug awareness courses to be able to talk to their children about drugs; and provide talks to young people.

Contact: Denise Godwin

Tel: 01273 698500

Funders: Safer Cities; Sussex Drug Prevention Team; Social Services

Needs assessment methods: Through a meeting with the Home Office and other statutory agencies, it became clear that there was a real need for an agency to provide the services that the Parent Drug Advice Network is offering.

Target group: Parents

Methods and evaluation: Parents' drug awareness courses run over two evenings or one day. They offer: a telephone answering machine service; telephone advice and information; home visits or office appointments; parents' self-help support groups; referral to other agencies; presentations/talks given at schools to parents/teachers; presentations to young people on drug issues; and sustained support to parents of drug-using young people.

User evaluation sheets are completed after courses by parents of young people, and plans are in hand for an independent evaluation.

SAME SKY

Wellesley House, 3–8 Waterloo Place, Brighton, East Sussex BN2 2NB

Tel: 01273 571106   **Fax:** 01273 606668

Contact: Pippa Smith

Health authority: East Sussex, Brighton and Hove

Other drug services: Community safety; arts activities targeted at vulnerable young people

Main business: Community/celebratory arts organisation

Detached and other drugs education work

This initative offers alternatives to drug use, and encouraged and helped organise a football session in the local leisure centre. Young unemployed males joined this for a 10-week programme. It encourages discussions about drugs, promotes harm reduction use on the estate, and provides advice and information.

Contact: Kim Breaks

Tel: 01273 571106

Funders: Youth Service; Drug Prevention Team

Needs assessment methods: A survey was carried out, as well as discussions with local residents, professionals and young people.

Target age groups: 11 and over

Target group: Neighbourhoods

Methods and evaluation: The project encourages alternative activities and has information available at all times in youth centres and from the detached team. It has established series of outing groups and offers an open club, where drugs issues can be discussed.

Staff write reports, and young people evaluate activities. If the activities are not instant, it is very difficult to get any commitment.

Strictly Seaside Project – Brighton

The project involved a site-specific dance activity, professionally led, for one hundred 16–25-year-olds. It was completed in July 1996.

Contact: Pippa Smith

Tel: 01273 571106

Partners: South East Arts; Brighton and Hove Borough Council; Brighton and Hove Drug Prevention Team

Funders: South East Arts; Brighton and Hove Borough Council, Drug Prevention Team

Target age group: 16–25

Target groups: School/college students

Methods: This project was primarily focused on the creation of costume, music and dance. The dance was new and 'experimental', but took place outside of the usual club atmosphere. The young people involved were exposed to a professional creative experience and a team which did not rely on drugs for its 'highs'.

UNIVERSITY OF BRIGHTON STUDENTS UNION (UBSU)

UBSU Cockcroft Building, Lewes Road, Brighton, East Sussex BN2 4GJ

Tel: 01273 642870   **Fax:** 01273 600694

Contact: Harvey Atkinson

Health authority: East Sussex, Brighton and Hove

Other drug services: Student drug education

Main business: Representation and empowerment of University of Brighton Students Union members

National Student Drug Education Project

The project provides camera-ready artwork to NUS-affiliated colleges to print drug education materials in their own union publications.

Contact: Dexter Coombe

Tel: 01273 722221

Partners: Sussex Drug Prevention Team; National Union of Students; UBSU; AIDS education project

Funders: Home Office Drug Prevention Initiative; UBSU

WOODINGDEAN YOUTH ADVICE AND INFORMATION

Hazel Cottage, Warren Road, Woodingdean, Brighton, East Sussex BN2 6DA

Tel: 01273 600606

Contact: Lynne Kealy

Health authority: East Sussex, Brighton and Hove

Other drug services: Community safety; training

Main business: Making contact with young people with a view to helping them to maximise their potential, and to increase their knowledge about lifestyle issues and their confidence to make informed decisions.

Mobile unit

The unit is involved in empowering young people by providing them with information regarding lifeskills and allowing them to develop the confidence and knowledge to make informed decisions.

Contact: Lynne Kealy

Tel: 01273 600606

Partners: Social Services: Youth Concern; school nurse; youth workers in the area

Funders: Woodingdean Youth Advice and Information; Social Services

Needs assessment methods: Qualitative research included: consultation with young people in schools and informal settings; and structured and unstructured interviews with young people, parents, teachers, and youth workers. Quantitative methods included surveys through the schools, the results of which indicated that drugs were considered less of a problem than they actually turned out to be.

Target age group: 11 and over

Target groups: Neighbourhoods

Methods and evaluation: Activities include: encouraging and facilitating youth projects, such as the building of a skateboard ramp and corresponding fund raising; providing alternative activities to drug taking; and setting up a parents' support group to educate parents about drugs and their misuse.

Evaluation is through feedback from various individuals.

YATA (YOUTH AND TRANQUILLIZER ADDICTION PROJECT)

TRANXACTION, 21b Prince Albert Street, Brighton, East Sussex BN1 1HF

Tel: 01273 329200

Contact: Jane McLoughlin

Health authority: East Sussex, Brighton and Hove

Other drug services: Treatment

Youth and Tranquillizer Addiction (YATA)

The project is based on the production of information leaflets for young people (under 25 years). It aims to raise awareness of the dangers of benzodiazepine misuse, when used alone or in conjunction with other drugs, e.g. alcohol. A leaflet also advertises Tranxaction's drop-in service to young people.

Contact: Jane McLoughlin

Tel: 01273 329200

Funders: Drug Prevention Team; Health Authority

Target age groups: 11–21

Target groups: Users of benzodiazepines; neighbourhoods

Methods: Pocket-sized leaflets, designed to be attractive to young people, are distributed via local agencies. Young people wanting further information, or already experiencing problems as a result of benzodiazepine misuse, are encouraged to seek further help from Tranxaction, whose drop-in service is promoted on the back of leaflets.

CROWBOROUGH YOUTH SERVICE

Youth Office, Beacon Community College, Beeches Road, Crowborough, East Sussex TN6 2AS

Tel: 01892 653451   **Fax:** 01892 663763

Contact: Adrian Parker

Health authority: East Sussex, Brighton and Hove

Main business: Working with young people in an informal manner – with the emphasis on educational participation through activities which young people attend in a voluntary capacity

Crowborough Youth Mobile Project

The project aimed to increase young people's knowledge on lifestyles issues, including drugs, and to increase their opportunities to develop positive, healthy and rewarding lives. This was achieved by operating a mobile youth information and advice unit in Crowborough and the surrounding rural areas, and seeking out young people in locations where they congregate. The project ended in July 1996.

Contact: Adrian Parker

Tel: 01892 653451

Partners: Social Services; Beacon Community College; Health Authority

Funders: Sussex Drug Prevention Team; Social Services, Beacon Community College; Health Authority

Needs assessment methods: A short statistical report was drawn up on the numbers of young people meeting. Recordings were made by discussion with young people who attended the local youth clubs and students at the college (qualitative evidence).

Target groups: Neighbourhoods; rural communities

Methods and evaluation: The project used the following methods: discussion groups; work with individuals; card packs; opinion games; board games, such as Mansworld and Time of the Month; Six Pack (games to increase awareness of drugs and alcohol); and interaction and dialogues.

Quantitative recording is intended, to: evaluate attendance, and repeat contacts and what was done on each evening. Qualitative recording will interview young people on their views of the mobile units and ask if the information/advice has affected attitudes and behaviour, increased knowledge, etc.

SEASIDE CENTRE – OUTREACH PROJECT ON THE EDGE

95 Seaside Road, Eastbourne, East Sussex BN21 3PL

Tel: 01323 412412   **Fax:** 01323 412412

Contacts: Alison Stanley, Nick Bolton

Health authority: East Sussex, Brighton and Hove

Other drug services: Treatment; community safety; training; counselling; sessional work; outreach support

Outreach work – On the Edge

The project involves building relationships with groups of young people, especially on the street, and educating and supporting young people involved in, or contemplating using or taking drugs.

Contact: Alison Stanley

Tel: 01323 412412

Funders: Joint finance; Comic Relief; Home Office, Health of the Nation

Needs assessment methods:

Questionnaires and informal group discussions with young people showed that: 45 per cent of young people between the ages of 15 and 20 had been offered and tried illegal drugs. Research also indicated that they needed help/support but would not come to the centre.

Target age groups: 11–21

Target groups: Not at school; homeless; neighbourhoods; groups

Methods and evaluation: The project is based on teamwork, informally educating young people through 'role model' education, using drama/role-plays, art work, information and a street work team. It aims to educate young people in a 'culture-friendly' way – using their language 'on their patch'.

Evaluation is mainly through team meetings and feedback, as well as looking at statistics and contact sheets which help to evaluate how successful the work is. Feedback sheets are being produced for the agencies/youth clubs visited.

YWCA OCKLYNGE YOUTH AND COMMUNITY CENTRE

Ocklynge Road, Eastbourne, East Sussex BN21 1PY

Tel: 01323 722924

Contact: Sue Relf

Health authority: East Sussex, Brighton and Hove

Main business: Community work, promoting family life and community spirit

Kids Plus

This is a Saturday afternoon of activities and fun for families (no unaccompanied children) at low cost to build relationships, promote family life, and educate parents and young people about drug misuse.

Contact: Sue Relf

Tel: 01323 733924

Partners: Health Authority Drug Liaison Team; Social Services Community Development; Eastbourne Borough Council Play Development

Funders: Sussex Drug Prevention Team; YWCA Ocklynge Youth and Community Centre

Needs assessment methods: The project was born out of Sussex Drugs Prevention Team criteria and research – 'Drug prevention in the community'.

Target groups: Parents (in particular families); neighbourhoods

CROWBOROUGH YOUNG PEOPLE'S WORKING GROUP

Social Services, 7 George Street, Hailsham, East Sussex BN27 1AD

Tel: 01323 841103   **Fax:** 01323 442305

Contact: Mal Cross

Health authority: East Sussex, Brighton and Hove

Advice and information mobile

The main aim of this pilot project is to increase young people's knowledge on lifestyle issues, including drugs, and to increase their opportunities to develop positive, healthy and rewarding lives. The project operates a mobile youth information and advice unit in Crowborough and the surrounding rural areas, seeking out young people in locations where they congregate.

Contact: Mal Cross

Tel: 01323 841103

Partners: Social Education workers; youth services; health services

Funders: Sussex Drug Prevention Team; Health Authority; East Sussex County Council; Beacon Community College, Wealden Social Services

Needs assessment methods: Quantitative and qualitative recordings are being carried out.

Target age groups: 11 and over

Target group: Rural communities

Methods: The project uses the following methods: to refer on where necessary; to interact with young people in groups or one-to-one; using specifically designed games and packs, and written information; to work in small social groups; to provide a mobile unit in a rural car park, which is frequented by young people, because they have nowhere to go; to adopt a community development approach which enables young community members in the area to set their own agenda and pace when they board the mobile; to provide a community focal point and a localised service; and to act as a co-supporting team of workers.

TRINITY PROJECT

6 Trinity Street, Hastings, East Sussex TN34 1HG

Tel: 01424 426375   **Fax:** 01424 722207

Contact: Nick Casey

Health authority: East Sussex, Brighton and Hove

Other drug services: Treatment; community safety; criminal justice; training; rural and urban outreach

Urban youth outreach

This project targets young people in the centre of Hastings – on the seafront, in the amusements, on the pier, in local nightclubs – to ensure that they are aware of the Trinity Project, and to provide information and harm minimisation.

Contact: Nick Casey

Tel: 01424 426375

Partners: Youth service; commercial organisations

Funder: Small members panel grant

Needs assessment methods: Contact with the service users and providers identified a need for the service.

Target age groups: 11 and over

Target group: Neighbourhoods

Methods and evaluation: The project works on the streets to identify young persons at risk, and then feeds them into the evening-opening session, where a range of interventions are used to enable the individual to firstly identify their goals, and then to work towards it. Interventions include Motivational Interviewing and solution-focused work, as well as offering a practical approach to the resolution of associated problems.

Evaluation is carried out by Simon Sandberg, the Department of Health and Peter Mason, Innovations group.

HOVE YMCA

17 Marmion Road, Hove, East Sussex BN3 5FS

Tel: 01273 731742   **Fax:** 01273 885565

Contacts: Don Brown, David Standing

Health authority: East Sussex, Brighton and Hove

Other drug services: Treatment; training

Main business: Youth and community work

Drug and Crime Prevention Project

The project aimed to build on the existing work of the YMCA with young people who were using illegal drugs, or who were at risk of using them. It targeted at-risk young people, and through identifying the underlying causes of use, tried to deal with the problems through group and one-to-one work, and by offering alternative activities and support systems. The project finished in March 1996.

Contact: Don Brown

Tel: 01273 731742

Partners: Police; youth advice centre; Social Services; churches; Education Welfare Office

Funders: Young People at Risk from Drugs (DoH grant scheme); Sussex Police Authority

Needs assessment methods: YMCA research showed that 58 per cent of 500 young people had used drugs. The research also showed anxiety and depression amongst drug users, suggesting that drug use is a symptom of other problems.

Target age groups: 11–18

Target groups: Offenders; not at school; homeless; parents; neighbourhoods; those at risk of drug use

Methods and evaluation: The project used the following methods: mentoring one-to-one support; outreach at local meeting places. Structured programmes, such as football training, trips and events, girls' groups and a 15+ coffee bar; and small group and individual mentoring using a holistic approach to life skills.

Evaluation is primarily though record keeping of an individual's progress by the mentor/keyworker. Performance targets are also set and evaluated by workers and there is a self–report completed by individual young people.

PASSWORD

212 High Street, Lewes, East Sussex BN7 2NH

Tel: 01273 473422   **Fax:** 01273 483109 **e-mail:** info@srcc.org.uk

Contact: Pat Buesnel

Health authority: East Sussex, Brighton and Hove

Main business: To promote, support and empower rural communities, rural people and community organisations in Sussex

Password – information/advice service

The project aims to take information and advice to young people (aged 13-18) living in the north Lewes district. The information focuses on health and related issues, including drugs. The project addresses rural isolation, poor transport and low levels of service by transporting information, advice and workers to locations where young people live.

Contact: Jo May

Tel: 01273 473422

Partner: Youth service

Funders: Social Services and Health Authority; Drug Prevention Initiative

Needs assessment methods: In 1994, a part-time worker and some volunteers carried out structured and informal interviews with 103 young people aged 13–18. It was found that 89.3 per cent had not used an information and advice service, but 85.5 per cent would if a local service were available. At the time they were most likely to turn to friends, parents or doctors for information and advice.

Target age groups: 13–18

Target group: Rural communities

Methods and evaluation: At present Password visits four villages. In two of them it meets once a week and offers recreational activities, information and materials. The workers are available for the young people to access. Also provided are issue-based activities to stimulate thought, discussion and learning. By taking part in developing the service, the young people also develop personal skills. In two other villages, Password is carrying out attached work and is in the early stages of developing the service.

Monitoring and evaluation is ongoing. Monitoring is done via nightly recording sheets including qualitative and quantitative data. Regular evaluation meetings are held with workers on the project. Lewes Joint Finance is monitoring the project along with the Drugs Prevention Initiative, who will be appointing outside evaluators. This will include the views of participants.

HAVEN YOUTH MOBILE

2c Meeching Road, Newhaven, East Sussex BN9 9XG

Tel: 01273 611396   **Fax:** 01273 612058

Contact: Jan Murphy

Health authority: East Sussex, Brighton and Hove

Main business: Informal education of young people

Haven Youth Mobile

The mobile offers a sexual health and drugs prevention service for young people.

Contact: Jan Murphy

Tel: 01273 611396

Partners: Drug Prevention Team; East Sussex, Brighton and Hove Health Authority; Family Health Services Authority; East Sussex Health Authority; Social Services; East Sussex County Council Adviser (Drugs)

Funders: Drug Prevention Team; youth service, Family Health Services Authority; East Sussex Health Authority

Needs assessment methods: Information from other research projects indicated a need for this service.

Target age groups: 11 and over

Methods: Two youth workers and a nurse staff a mobile unit. These workers engage in discussion with young people and play games which are about sex education, alcohol and drug use. Young people are shown how to use condoms, and condoms are supplied free of charge.

PEACEHAVEN HOUSE PROJECT

168 South Coast Road, Peacehaven, East Sussex BN10 8JH

Tel: 01273 582467

Contact: Mark Mansbridge

Health authority: East Sussex, Brighton and Hove

Community Youth Peer Education Project

Through street work, the project drew together a group who discussed drug and sexual health/lifestyle issues, created a pack of information cards and used them in peer education.

Contact: Harry Nicholson

Tel: 01273 582467

Partner: Lewes Youth Service

Funders: Weavers Benevolent; Tudor Trust; Home Office Drug Prevention Initiative

Needs assessment methods: Extensive research including street work and questionnaires, produced a full report, including prioritised needs.

Target age groups: 11 and over

Target group: Neighbourhoods

Methods: In addition to information cards, the project youth worker is developing a drop-in social space in a local community house, information and support to young people, and a range of summer activities – barbecues, etc. Street outreach is also ongoing.

West Sussex

PLeAD (PARENTS LEARNING ABOUT DRUGS)

Crawley Drug Advice Centre, The Tree (Annexe), 103 High Street, Crawley, West Sussex RH10 1DD

Tel: 01293 548350   **Fax:** 01403 256184

Contact: Jim Noton

Health authority: West Sussex

Other drug services: Community safety; training; educating parents

Parents Learning About Drugs

This initiative offers free training for parents to gain a knowledge and understanding of the drug culture, and the confidence and skills that will enable them to talk about drugs within their own families.

Contact: Jim Noton

Tel: 01293 548350

Partners: Crawley Drug Advice Centre; youth service; Sussex Drug Prevention Team

Funders: Home Office; Round Table; Sun Alliance; CIBA Pharmaceuticals, youth service

Target group: Parents

Methods and evaluation: The training is in groups no larger than 20 over one session lasting two hours. This is divided into two modules: the first with the aim of imparting drugs information, the second for enhancing parenting skills. Group work is preferred, as well as an emphasis on experiential learning and participative learning. The project aims to reach as many parents as possible and use whatever channels are available to reach them.

Continual evaluation is carried out by trainers at regular meetings as well as through response forms.

PARENT NETWORK SUSSEX

The Old Rectory, East Marden, Near Chichester, West Sussex PO18 9JE

Tel: 01243 535208   **Fax:** 01243 535208

Contact: Linda Connell

Health authority: West Sussex

Other drug services: Parent support

Main business: Providing groups for educating parents in communication, and offering support for families

Supporting and empowering parents

This initiative provides training in groups for parents and for anyone living or working with children in which new strategies and communication skills are developed, particularly that of listening.

Contact: Linda Connell

Tel: 01798 831715

Funders: Arlemic Trust; Bernard Leer Foundation; Tudor Trust

Target groups: Parents

Methods and evaluation: The initiative uses experiential learning, in which a specific topic is discussed at each 2½ hour session. A booklet is provided for each session, and the group is strongly encouraged to continue to meet when the sessions are over.

Evaluation is carried out by Dr Hilton Davis, Consultant Psychologistat, Guy's Hospital. In addition there are 10 parent link groups, and 10 control groups.

REACHOUT – RURAL YOUTH MOBILE BUS

Media House, Pound Street, Petworth, West Sussex GU28 0DX

Tel: 01798 342547   **Fax:** 01798 342547

Contact: Maureen Sargent

Health authority: West Sussex

Other drug services: Training

Main business: Youth service to rural areas

West Sussex Rural Youth Mobile Project

The bus provides a youth service, information and a social venue in villages with little or no active youth provision.

Contact: Maureen Sargent

Tel: 01798 342547

Partners: West Sussex County Council; Sussex Rural Community Council

Funders: West Sussex County Council, Crime Prevention; Drug Prevention initiative; West Sussex Health Authority; Horsham District Council, Sussex police; Foundation for Sports and the Arts; Body Shop

Needs assessment methods: A survey of existing services and facilities highlighted the gaps within rural areas. Discussions with individual parish councils and local groups helped to define the need.

Target age groups: 11–18

Target group: Rural communities

Methods: The bus carries information, leaflets, multi-media-based information, resources (games, etc.) to help educate and inform about drugs and their use. The ReachOut Project has a team of peer trainers who are themselves trained by West Sussex Health Authority. The project is also developing arts-based work which will supplement existing activities. It provides a social centre where young people can find out about, discuss and seek help about drugs if necessary.

Tyne and Wear

NORTHUMBRIA DRUGS PREVENTION TEAM

Lombard House, 4-8 Lombard Street, Newcastle-Upon-Tyne, Tyne and Wear NE1 3AE

Tel: 0191 233 1972   **Fax:** 0191 233 1973

Contact: Jayne Moules

Health authority: Newcastle and North Tyneside

NE Choices drugs prevention programme

The programme was a multi-model drugs prevention intervention employing social marketing theory, designed to prevent or delay the onset of drug use among young people and to encourage family and schools to communicate with them on drugs issues. It ran from January to March 1996.

Contact: Jayne Moules

Tel: 0191 233 1972

Partners: All six local authorities in Tyne and Wear

Funders: Home Office Drug Prevention Initiative; Procter and Gamble

Needs assessment methods: Interviews of focus groups by Teesside University revealed that 13-year-old children were those most likely to be offered drugs.

Target age group: 11–16

Target groups: Parents; neighbourhoods

Methods and evaluation: A drama workshop was run by Northern Stage and funded by Drug Prevention Initiative at 17 selected schools throughout Northumbria for one week each. One session was held with each class of Year 9 pupils, with a summary session at the end, and an interactive session held with their parents. A magazine funded by Procter and Gamble was sent to about 80 per cent of 13-year-olds in the region. Community awareness was raised during the workshops.

Evaluation was through a questionnaire provided with the magazine. The NE Choices programme served as a pilot for a three-year programme that commenced in January 1997. Strathclyde University will evaluate this programme.

UNEW (UNIVERSITY OF NEWCASTLE-UPON-TYNE)

1 Yankerville Terrace, Jesmond, Newcastle-Upon-Tyne, Tyne and Wear NE2 3AH

Tel: 0191 232 5131   **Fax:** 0191 2816 591

Health authority: Newcastle and North Tyneside

Other drug services: Training

Main business: Child and adolescent mental health

Prevention of drug use among boys

The project centred on boys with disruptive behaviour, and involved identifying boys (11–14 years) in comprehensive schools with behaviour disorders, according to teachers. These were randomised to two different universities for multi-modal intervention. The aim was the prevention of drug use in those boys vulnerable to abuse. The project finished in March 1996, and subsequently gathered follow-up data.

Contact: Paul McArdle

Tel: 0191 232 5131

Partners: Local Education Authority; Regional Drug and Alcohol Service

Funders: Department of Health; Local Education Authority, Newcastle City Health Trust

Needs assessment methods: The need was based on earlier surveys of substance use in young people.

Target groups: Males; parents

Methods and evaluation: The intervention made use of: small-group education in basics; individual counselling; informal social skills; and drug education.

Evaluation is through questionnaires for parents, teachers and youths, with non-intervention control.

COMMUNITY ADDICTION TEAM

11 Norfolk Street, Sunderland, Tyne and Wear SR1 1EA

Tel: 0191 510 8933   **Fax:** 0191 565 4910

Contact: Chris Laydon

Health authority: Sunderland

Other drug services: Treatment; training; HIV promotion; day care; outreach; clinical services

A19 drop-in

This is a confidential advice and information centre for young people that provides access to harm reduction/risk minimisation information in the community, and the opportunity for primary prevention and to develop a detached youth work team.

Contact: Suzanne Byrne

Tel: 0191 510 8933

Partners: Community Addiction Team; Pennywell Neighbourhood Centre; Pennywell Youth Project

Funders: Local authority (Drugs Accord); Health Authority, Children In Need

Target age groups: 11–21

Target groups: Neighbourhoods; community groups

Methods: The centre has adapted health service protocols, etc., for a community setting. It also: liaises and networks with community groups, including schools; provides resources and expertise; and trains and supports youth workers in specific recognition, assessment and intervention skills.

Young People's Support Service (YPSS)

The service provides easy access to addiction agencies for young people within the youth justice system, Social Services residential accommodation, and young women's refuges.

Contact: Suzanne Byrne

Tel: 0191 510 8933

Partners: Social Services; youth justice; women's refuge; residential homes; family support team; carers centre

Funder: Priority Health Care, Wearside

Needs assessment methods: An initial outreach networking and community liaison exercise revealed a need for accessible services for young people.

Target groups: Offenders; parents

Methods and evaluation: Methods used include: advice and information using a harm minimisation approach; collaborative work with young people; training workers and carers; advocacy support for workers; user-friendly, safe, non-judgemental environment in which to enhance peer awareness of community drug issues.

There is a continuous evaluation through monthly reports, internal evaluation, internal qualitative assessment forms, user surveys and anecdotal reports.

COMMUNITY EDUCATION SERVICE

Monkwearmouth Hospital, Newcastle Road, Sunderland, Tyne and Wear SR5 1NB

Tel: 0191 565 6256   **Fax:** 0191 569 9248

Contact: Tanya Sherriff

Health authority: Sunderland

Main business: Providing statutory and voluntary youth provision and community education

The Buzz Network peer education projects

The project aims: to empower young people, through participation, to examine issues around drug use/misuse; and to increase their communication skills and knowledge base, enabling them to empower their peers and pass on factual information.

Contact: Tanya Sherriff

Tel: 0191 565 6256

Partners: Community education; youth service

Funders: Single Regeneration Budget (part of Sunderland City Council's anti-drug strategy); Strategic Initiative Budget via the Sunderland City Drugs Accord.

Target age group: 11–16

Evaluation: Residential weekends form the basis of evaluation. Diaries have been designed to evaluate how many young people the peer educators are reaching.

THE BASE

26 Esplanade, Whitley Bay, Tyne and Wear NE26 2AS

Tel: 0191 253 2127   **Fax:** 0191 253 3195

Contact: Richard Taylor

Health authority: Newcastle and North Tyneside

Other drug services: Treatment; diversionary activities

Detached youth work and peer education

The aim of the work with young people on the streets, using confidence building and skill development, was to enable peer education to be developed. The main project ran until March 1996, though some work continues with additional funding.

Contact: Richard Taylor

Tel: 0191 253 2127

Partner: North Tyneside Community Services

Funder: Young People at Risk from Drugs (DoH grant scheme); Single Regeneration Budget funds via North Tyneside Council

Target age groups: 11 and over

Target groups: Offenders; homeless; children in care; neighbourhoods; arcade users

Evaluation: Evaluation was through questionnaires, discussion, informal analysis, visiting the evaluator, and monitoring forms.

West Midlands

ALLENS CROFT PROJECT

44 Allens Croft Road, Kings Heath, Birmingham, West Midlands B14 6RQ

Tel: 0121 444 4897   **Fax:** 0121 624 6323

Contacts: Fred Rattley/Ged Lodge

Health authority: Birmingham

Main business: Neighbourhood community project – youth work, economic development, and community development

Mobile health project

Using a specially converted vehicle and a team of detached youth workers, the project made contact with young people on the streets of Brandwood, Birmingham. The project finished in March 1997.

Contact: Ged Lodge

Tel: 0121 444 4897

Partner: Birmingham Youth Service

Funder: Health Authority

Needs assessment methods: Interviews were recorded with and questionnaires completed by young people on the streets.

Target age groups: 11–21

Target groups: Not at school; parents

Methods and evaluation: Youth workers met with groups of young people on the streets and set up informal discussion groups using a wide range of resources, e.g. leaflets, quizzes, and drugs care. They also offered organisations as referral points. The project also worked with one group to produce a video around a drug prevention theme which was funded by the Drugs Prevention Initiative.

A log book is kept, together with individual case studies and monitoring sheets. Group activities are also evaluated by participants using both written resources and oral statements through video interviews.

PARENTS FOR PREVENTION

St Vincent's Hall, Botany Walk, Birmingham, West Midlands B16 8ED

Tel: 0121 454 5805   **Fax:** 0121 454 9259

Contact: Rosie Higgins

Health authority: Birmingham

Other drug services: Parents' information; education; support service

Drug awareness talks

The talks aim: to raise awareness of drugs – their effects, methods and reasons for use, and signs and symptoms; to explore ways in which parents can educate their children about drugs; to identify strategies for coping should problems arise through drug use; and to inform parents of local support agencies.

Contact: Rosie Higgins

Tel: 0121 454 5805

Partners: Police; drug agencies; Local Education Authority; Health Education Unit

Funder: Drug Prevention Team

Needs assessment methods: Networking with policy makers, service providers and the community (especially parents) highlighted the gaps in provision for parents who generally feel ill-informed and ill-equipped to educate their children about drugs.

Target groups: Parents; neighbourhoods; community groups; rural communities

Methods and evaluation: The talks facilitate discussion, using a variety of activities, e.g. card games, brainstorms, questionnaires, use of slides/video snippets, and whole/small group discussions. Occasionally guest speakers sit on a panel for question-and-answer sessions.

Evaluation is by pre- and post-session questionnaire/informal standard questions.

Helpline and befriending service

The service aims to provide information, advice and support to parents concerned about their child's drug use, and to help parents to tap into other support agencies, as and where appropriate.

Contact: Rosie Higgins

Tel: 0121 454 5805

Partners: Variety of agencies

Funders: Drug Prevention Team; TSB; British Telecom

Needs assessment methods: Networking with policy makers, service providers and the community (especially parents) highlighted the fact that many parents of under 16-year-olds are reluctant to turn to statutory agencies for support, and feel that community drug agencies who deal with 'addicts' are inappropriate for this age group.

Target age groups: 11 and over

Target groups: Parents (any parent/guardian)

Methods and evaluation: The helpline is usually the first point of contact for parents wanting information and advice. Each caller is sent an information pack tailor-made to suit their particular situation. Those parents requiring ongoing support are offered an appointment with a befriender at a venue of their choice (usually in the home). The befriender will provide a listening ear and offer advice as appropriate. Referrals may be made to specialist agencies if required and the befriender will act as a mediator if requested. Support groups are formed as/when there are several parents who express an interest in meeting with others experiencing similar problems.

Quantitative data are collected on the number of calls, as well as the time and nature of the calls, to help inform the development of all the services. A process for collecting qualitative information from clients is being developed.

Living with Teenagers programme

The programme aims to educate parents by raising awareness, providing information and developing skills on the topic of parenting teenagers.

Contact: Rosie Higgins

Tel: 0121 454 5805

Partner: North Birmingham College

Funders: North Birmingham College; Cadburys

Needs assessment methods: Various discussions took place: with parents attending drug awareness talks; with schools in identifying parents' concerns; and with Norlink staff on the programme development.

Target group: Parents

Methods and evaluation: The programme comprises a 10-week accredited course (half a day a week) or tailor-made sessions ranging from two to six hours. The sessions use a combination of facilitated input and group work to explore the issues relating to living with teenagers. Emphasis is on skills development and problem-solving techiques. At the end of each course, parents are invited to attend a bi-monthly support session.

Evaluation is by individual pre-/post-course questionnaires and informal discussion.

UNIVERSITY OF BIRMINGHAM GUILD OF STUDENTS

Edgbaston Park Road, Edgbaston, Birmingham, West Midlands B15 2TU

Tel: 0121 472 1841   **Fax:** 0121 471 1563

Contact: Steve Sanger

Health authority: Birmingham

Main business: Student union

Making Informed Choices

This is a drugs education scheme that aims to measure, evaluate and prevent the use of drugs by students at the University of Birmingham. It is coupled with a non-judgemental approach to education on the subject.

Contact: Steve Sanger

Tel: 0121 472 1841

Partners: Drug Prevention Team; student support and counselling centre

Funders: Home Office Drug Prevention

Initiative; University of Birmingham

Target age groups: 17–21

Target group: Students

Methods and evaluation: The project educates via club-type flyers, professional posters, a travelling workshop-based play, student radio, student clubs, student interface, information on the Campus Super Highway, links with sports teams, and information stalls in the student union.

DUDLEY DRUGS EDUCATION FOR YOUNG PEOPLE

8 Parson Street, Dudley, West Midlands DY1 1JJ

Tel: 01384 453191   **Fax:** 01384 453189

Contact: Dewi Williams

Health authority: Dudley

Other drug services: Training

Main business: Youth and community work

Drama Drugs Prevention

The programme catered for individual group needs, and was delivered through a comprehensive package, including drama strategies and a resource pack. It finished in April 1997.

Contact: Anette O'Reilly

Tel: 01384 453191

Partner: Birmingham and Black Country Drug Prevention Team

Funders: Birmingham and Black Country Drug Prevention Team; Community Development Unit

Target groups: Indian; Pakistani; Bangladeshi; not at school; homeless; children in care; parents; neighbourhoods

Methods: Direct training was given through the employment of specific drama strategies for volunteer group needs.

Dudley Drugs Education for Young People

After completing a needs analysis with both youth workers and young people, a curriculum model of drugs education was developed that could be implemented in a variety of informal situations.

Contact: Dewi Williams

Tel: 01384 453191

Partners: Birmingham and Black Country Drug Prevention Team; The Warehouse (Voluntary Dudley Drugs Project)

Funders: Birmingham and Black Country Drug Prevention Team; Dudley Borough, Department for Education and Employment grants for education support and training (GEST).

Needs assessment methods: A need was identified following informal discussions with youth workers and young people.

SALTWELLS EDUCATION DEVELOPMENT CENTRE

Bowling Green Road, Netherton, Dudley, West Midlands DY2 9LY

Tel: 01384 813776   **Fax:** 01384 410436

Contact: Irene Hayes

Health authority: Dudley

Other drug services: Training; awareness raising in the community

Parent/Children Opening the Dialogue

This forum takes place in two sessions, held over two evenings: first – information/awareness raising with parents only; and second – parents and children together expressing fears/concerns and needs.

Contact: Irene Hayes

Tel: 01384 813776

Partners: Education welfare officers; teachers; police; youth workers

Funder: Health Authority

Target age groups: 11–16

Target group: Parents (through Parent–Teacher Association)

Methods: Evening 1: parents meet and discuss concerns and fears. Information is given through video, leaflets/quiz and trainer input. Parents in groups discuss case studies relating to coping with a child who is misusing substances. Evening 2: for parents and children of all ages (mixed family groups). The evening starts with a fun quiz, with team names/running totals/prizes, etc., and the second half of the evening is parent-only groups.

CASCADE – SOLIHULL PEER EDUCATION DRUG PROGRAMME

Keepers Lodge, Chelmsley Road, Chelmsley Wood, Solihull, West Midlands B37 7UA

Tel: 0121 788 3436   **Fax:** 0121 779 7093 **e-mail:** lenmack@leam.u-net.com

Contacts: Len Mackin, Helen Thompson

Health authority: Solihull

Other drug services: Community; training; work with parent groups

Cascade

CASCADE is a young persons' peer-led drug education programme that works with young people aged 11–25. Young people are trained and supported in developing programmes to keep young people safe.

Contacts: Len Mackin, Helen Thompson

Tel: 0121 788 3436

Partners: Solihull Local Education Authority; Solihull Health Promotion Unit/Service; Solihull Health Authority

Funders: Solihull Health Authority; Department for Education and Employment; Lynbury; Crime Prevention; Marks and Spencer

Needs assessment methods: The programme is based on the needs expressed by young people and volunteers. Drug Action Team groups feed into the process.

Target age groups: 11 and over

Target groups: Children in care; parents (through Parent–Teacher Association); community groups; rural communities, through Council for Voluntary Service networks

Methods and evaluation: Volunteers (under 25 years) are trained by CASCADE. They come from schools, colleges and the community, and after training go to work in venues such as schools, workshops, displays and roadshows. There are also 'on site' groups linked to a specific organisation. Other young people get involved for specific activities, e.g. art design for leaflets and materials.

Evaluation was carried out by: Solihull Health 1995/6 GEST Evaluation, and the Home Office 1994 – CDPU independent evaluation. Other evaluation is through research with participants and interviews with key agency personnel.

WALKWAYS – WALSALL YOUTH PROJECTS

Littleton Street Youth Club, Littleton Street West, Walsall, West Midlands WS1 2EQ

Tel: 01922 615393   **Fax:** 01922 28593

Contact: Alan Jarvis

Health authority: Walsall

Other drug services: Community safety; training; detached and outreach work

Illicit drugs outreach work

The aim of the work is to raise illicit drug awareness for both users and non-users, and to reduce the harm related to illicit drugs use.

Contact: Alan Jarvis

Tel: 01922 615393

Funders: Drug Prevention Initiative; Comic Relief; City Challenge

Target age groups: 11 and over

Target groups: Offenders; homeless; neighbourhoods

Methods: At present the drugs project is involved in contacting young people who do not have involvement with any other statutory or voluntary organisation. The venues for such activities are varied, ranging from street work to nightclubs.

The project is also involved in initiating two pieces of group work: an arts and multi-media group in conjunction with Jubilee Arts, the main aim of which is to create a CD-ROM for use in schools and youth centres aimed at raising drug awareness and highlighting some key issues from the young persons' perspective: and secondly, providing assistance to ex-users who want to start up a users/ex-users support group. Walkways act as a facilitator for the first few meetings and then withdraw and act only as a point of reference. Also, as and when requested, Walkways operate a training and education programme for schools and youth groups, as well as internal and external staff training.

SANDWELL COMMUNITY DRUG/ALCOHOL TEAM

Edward Street Hospital, West Bromwich, West Midlands B70 8NY

Tel: 0121 607 3440   **Fax:** 0121 607 3576

Contacts: Ken Stringer, Chris Stickler

Health authority: Sandwell

Other drug services: Treatment; community safety; criminal justice; training

Development of interactive CD-ROM

The CD-ROM will provide an educative facility for youth and parents incorporating young people's views on drug use and harm reduction information. The development process itself is geared to provide skills and to empower young people to present their own views.

Contact: Ken Stringer

Tel: 0121 607 3440

Partners: Drug Prevention Initiative; Jubilee Arts

Funders: Health authority; Drug Prevention Initiative

Target age groups: 11–18

Target groups: Not at school; homeless; children in care; parents; neighbourhoods; community groups

Methods: The project is still at the pilot stage, but it is envisaged that the ideas and views of local youth will be incorporated in order to appeal to this age group and to inform parents of the views held by young people.

Drug education

This education is based on discussion groups with young people, through which workers aim: to identify views held by young people, and to correct misinformation/provide information; to identify the variety and extent of young people's drug use; and to empower youth to take part in service planning.

Contact: Ken Stringer

Tel: 0121 607 3440

Partners: Youth services; peer education (sexual health) project

Funder: Health Authority

Target age groups: 11–18

Target groups: Black Caribbean; black African; black other; not at school

Methods: The approach has developed from providing a general information-giving service, to developing specific focus/task oriented groups and addressing particular issues around drugs, e.g. safety advice on use; effects on later life, etc. Issues are identified by youths themselves and groups are developed on request.

Juvenile justice link worker

The worker provides a drug service for young people passing through Sandwell's juvenile justice system. The aim is to co-ordinate an education and support network for workers involved with young people.

Contact: Chris Stickler

Tel: 0121 607 3440

Partners: Juvenile Justice Unit; Community Alternative for Young Offenders; Anchor Project

Funders: Health Authority; Drug Prevention Initiative

Needs assessment methods: The service arose from a young persons' drug-use survey carried out in Sandwell

Target age groups: 11–21

Target groups: Offenders

Methods: The project provides education regarding drugs and drug use with a harm minimisation approach. It is envisaged that drug education will be incorporated into supervision orders, and serve as an alternative to custody programmes. The project will also explore links between drug use and crime. Theatre and drama will be used, and possibly an interactive media project with Jubilee Arts based in West Bromwich.

Parents awareness group

The aim of the group is: to enable parents and youths to communicate more effectively regarding drug users; to provide youths with an understanding of the parental position; and to provide adults with some knowledge of youth views.

Contact: Ken Stringer

Tel: 0121 607 3440

Funders: Fundraising; Drug Prevention Initiative

Needs assessment methods: The group arose after a Sandwell youth drug-use survey.

Target groups: Not at school; parents; neighbourhoods

Methods: Groups were established through joint events involving a GP, education, a community drugs team, police and the youth service. Parents then organised themselves into locality based groups with a view to self-education. This went on to include improving communication between the youths and parents.

Safe Hands Ltd outreach work

This initiative aims to provide information from an outreach perspective to young people concerning the use of drugs to help them to stop or minimise drug use.

Contact: Roy McFarlane

Tel: 0121 555 6696

Partners: Drug Prevention Initiative; Community Safety Team/Unit

Funders: Drug Prevention Initiative; Community Safety Team/Unit

Target age groups: 11 and over

North Yorkshire

THE PAVEMENT PROJECT – NORTHALLERTON DETACHED YOUTH WORK

Community House, Room 3b, 10 South Parade, Northallerton, North Yorkshire DL7 8SE

Tel: 01609 771971

Contact: Heather Corcoran

Health authority: North Yorkshire

Main business: Working with young people on any issues that affect their lives

Residential project – Carlton Challenge

The project involved taking young people on a residential experience to an outdoor activity centre in March 1996 to try out alternative activities to drug taking.

Contact: Heather Corcoran

Tel: 01609 771971

Partners: Community Education; Carlton Lodge Centre

Funder: The Pavement Project

Target age groups: 11–18

Methods and evaluation: The project was a 'Krypton Factor'-type weekend where the young people represented the Northallerton area in many competitive activities, both mental and physical (including visual arts, sport and theatre).

Questionnaires were completed by participants.

South Yorkshire

BAAS – BARNSLEY ALCOHOL ADVISORY SERVICE

8 Eastgate, Barnsley, South Yorkshire S70 2EX

Tel: 01226 779066

Contact: Simon Weldon

Health authority: Barnsley

Other drug services: Treatment; criminal justice; training; probation liaison project

Detached work project

The project aimed to provide a diversion from drugs for young people on the periphery of drug use; as well as for drug misusers. It finished in July 1996.

Contact: Denise Staples

Tel: 01226 753406

Funders: Police; Barnsley community

Needs assessment methods: Research project on young people's knowledge of drugs in a local secondary school revealed that young people want information, but not classroom teaching, and that not all young people attend youth centres.

Target age groups: 11–18

Target groups: Offenders; parents; neighbourhoods

Evaluation: This was carried out by Barnsley Community Resources, and was based on the number of contacts (basic, maintained and developed).

Drug Shout workshops

These provided drugs education and awareness training for parents and school children. They finished in February 1996.

Contact: Denise Staples

Tel: 01226 753406

Partners: Wombwell High School; Darfield Falston School

Funders: South Yorkshire Police; Barnsley Metropolitan City Council

Needs assessment methods: Informal street interviews which were carried out in 1994 by detached workers looking at the best way to address issues around drugs with young people showed that young people wanted information, but not in a classroom situation.

Target age group: 11–16

Target groups: Parents; governors; teachers

Methods and evaluation: The workshops addressed bullying and issues around drugs through role-play.

Young people's thoughts and needs were surveyed prior to the project, and their learning surveyed post project.

BARNSLEY COMMUNITY RESOURCES

Berneslai Close, Barnsley, South Yorkshire S70 2HS

Tel: 01226 770770   **Fax:** 01226 773599

Contact: Brigid Kane

Health authority: Barnsley

Other drug services: Community safety; training; information and counselling

Main business: Youth service, adult education and community development

Crown Estate Youth Action, Cudworth

The aim is to offer practical projects for young people aged 8–19 years.

Contact: David Hudson

Tel: 01226 753406

Partners: Crown Estate Parent and Toddler Group; Crown Estate Tenants and Residents Association; South Yorkshire Police; Barnsley Metropolitan Borough Council Leisure Service; Barnsley Metropolitan Borough Council Housing

Funders: Barnsley City Challenge; Barnsley Community Resources

Needs assessment methods:
A questionnaire and discussion group with young people ascertained the good and bad aspects of the estate and young people's current activities.

Target age groups: 8–19

Target groups: Parents; neighbourhoods; community groups

Dearne Substance Misuse Project

This project has fitted out a room in a local youth club for use by the substance misuse group.

Contact: Denise Staples

Tel: 01226 753406

Partners: Barnsley Health Authority Substance Misuse Team; probation

Funders: South Yorkshire Police Community Initiative

Target age groups: 11–18

Target groups: Users of anabolic steroids; neighbourhoods

Outreach work with young people

This work involves youth crime prevention initiatives based on the personal and social development of young people in three locations: the town centre, Athersley and Kendray.

Contact: Andy Fleming

Tel: 01226 771818

Partners: Schools; Crime Prevention Partnership

Funders: Single Regeneration Budget 1; Barnsley Metropolitan Borough Council; South Yorkshire Police

Target age groups: 11–21

Target groups: Not at school; neighbourhoods

Evaluation: This is be carried out by an independent organisation and funder, from feedback from young people, both formal and informal, which determines whether the aims and objectives have been met.

Project 4 x 4

The project offers a range of diversionary activities in Landrovers (off-road); and is used by Social Services, Probation and Community Resources.

Contact: Mandy Chester-Bristow

Tel: 01226 748822

Partners: Spectrum 4 x 4

Funders: Single Regeneration Budget 1; Spectrum 4 x 4

Needs assessment methods: This was assessed by an inter-agency form.

Target age groups: 11–21

Target groups: Offenders; not at school; homeless; children in care; neighbourhoods; community groups

Methods: The project is non-specific, and the issues and participants are identified by the users/purchasers of the service.

Single Regeneration Budget Outdoor Adventure Project

This project involves diversion activity, outdoor adventure and personal development.

Contact: Chris Spencer

Tel: 01226 742638

Partners: Barnsley Education Business Partnership; GAZ Project, Grimesthorpe

Funders: Single Regeneration Budget 1; Barnsley Metropolitan Borough Council

Needs assessment methods: A consultation exercise with existing providers identified a gap in provisions.

Target age groups: 11–18

Target groups: Offenders; not at school; neighbourhoods

Evaluation: This is carried out by TACADE and the Local Education Authority. There is also a questionnaire.

Youth Action Against Crime

This initiative has developed specific activities to give young people alternatives to crime (resulting from contacts with young people who use the streets as a recreational resource). The project finished in March 1997.

Contact: Denise Staples

Tel: 01226 753406

Funders: Dearne City Challenge; Barnsley, Doncaster and Rotherham youth services

Needs assessment methods: City Challenge undertook a major area-based community priority services survey (Sheffield Hallam University) which covered a range of issues, not just drugs.

Target age groups: 11–18

Target groups: Neighbourhoods

Evaluation: This is by interim report and user surveys.

YISS (Youth Information and Support Service)

This service provides advice and counselling for young people on all subjects, including drugs and alcohol.

Contact: Jill Rodger

Tel: 01226 299222

Funders: Barnsley City Challenge; Barnsley Community Resources

Target age groups: 11 and over

Target groups: Homeless; parent support group

Methods and evaluation: The service offers counsellors, one-to-one and group sessions; and also holds anonymous question sessions.

Evaluation is carried out by a borough-wide community education officer, OFSTED

BEECHURST HOSTEL FOR HOMELESS YOUNG PERSONS

189 Sheffield Road, Barnsley, South Yorkshire S70 4DE

Tel: 01226 296021

Contact: Sue Mellor

Health authority: Barnsley

Main business: Providing accommodation for homeless young people

Beechurst youth counselling service

The service develops projects to promote personal and social development and to assist in drugs rehabilitation.

Contact: Helen Murphy

Tel: 01226 296021

Funders: Single Regeneration Budget 1; Barnsley Health Authority; charitable trusts

Target age groups: 17 and over

Target groups: Offenders; homeless; children in care

Methods: The central focus of the service is counselling work, with an emphasis on guidance, training and helping young people to reach their potential (self-development).

YMCA BARNSLEY

8 Market Street, Hoyland, Barnsley, South Yorkshire S70 9QR

Tel: 01226 351414

Contact: Paula Taylor-McColl

Health authority: Barnsley

Hoyland 'Y' Project

This is a detached youth work project.

Contact: Paula Taylor-McColl

Tel: 01226 351414

Partners: Barnsley Metropolitan Borough Council Community Resources; South Yorkshire Police (community constables); Barnsley Metropolitan Borough Council Social Services; Barnsley National Health Trust; local schools

Funders: South Yorkshire Police Community Initiatives; Rotherham YMCA; NatWest Bank

Needs assessment methods: Informal interviews and questionnaires with young people revealed a lack of facilities for 14–17-year-olds locally, and the need for a local place to meet.

Target age groups: 11 and over

Target groups: Children in care; parents; community groups; rural communities

Methods and evaluation: This is very much a detached 'get out and see the people' project.

Output evaluation is by seeing what aims and objectives were met, and process evaluation is by examination of comprehensive project records.

GAZ – GRIMETHORPE ACTIVITY ZONE

The Acorn Centre, Grimethorpe, South Yorkshire S72 7BB

Tel: 01226 713599   **Fax:** 01226 781156

Contact: Andy Clow

Health authority: Barnsley

Main business: Youth and community work

Grimethorpe Activity Zone Project

This is a project for young people which addresses disaffection and drug misuse, aiming to reduce the incidence and prevalence of drug misuse amongst 10–25-year-olds in a deprived former mining village.

Contact: Andy Clow

Tel: 01226 713599

Partners: NACRO; Grimethorpe Partnership; South Yorkshire Police; Barnsley Social Services; Barnsley Community Resources; Carlton Bricks

Funders: Single Regeneration Budget 1; Barnsley Metropolitan Borough Council; Save the Children Fund; Getty Fund

Needs assessment methods: Consultation with young people in schools and informal settings used qualitative research – structured and unstructured interviews with young people, parents, teachers, youth workers; and quantitative research – surveys through schools to ascertain public perception of drug misuse.

Target age groups: 10–25

Target groups: Offenders; not at school; homeless; children in care; neighbourhoods

Methods and evaluation: The project uses informal educational methods, experiential learning and group work – reflecting on the past and thinking about the future. It also uses street work.

SCODA administered the funding for the project for the first year, and it was evaluated by Dr Simon Sandberg. Other evaluation procedures are: one-to-one informal interviewing; personal profile; comment forms; working interviews; and statistics of attendance, e.g. for detox.

NACRO – NEIGHBOURHOOD DEVELOPMENT UNIT

The Acorn Centre, 51 High Street, Grimethorpe, South Yorkshire S72 7BB

Tel: 01226 780795   **Fax:** 01226 781156

Contact: Linda Finney

Health authority: Barnsley

Other drug services: Community safety; criminal justice; training; welfare rights

Main business: Crime prevention and community safety through community development

Grimethorpe Neighbourhood Development Project

The project offers advice, support and community development, with an emphasis on prevention of re-offending and helping people to stop taking drugs.

Contact: Linda Finney

Tel: 01226 780795

Partners: Barnsley Community Resources; Social Services; South Yorkshire Police

Funders: Single Regeneration Budget 1; European Social Fund

Needs assessment methods: Qualitative research was carried out with (potential) users.

Target groups: Offenders; not at school; homeless; parents (referred by agencies); neighbourhoods; community groups

Methods and evaluation: Participants are referred by agencies and the evaluation is carried out by the manager and senior probation officer by talking to the different agencies worked with, hard data, and talking to users.

SHED

117 Rockingham Street, Sheffield, South Yorkshire S1 4EB

Tel: 0114 272 9164

Contacts: Susie Sykes/Anna Christophorou

Health authority: Sheffield

Other drug services: Treatment; Criminal justice

Counselling for young drug users

The project workers have a case load made up of young people who are experiencing problems as a result of recreational or experimental drug use.

Contact: Anna Christophorou

Tel: 0114 272 9164

Funders: Single Regeneration Budget; Police Authority; Regional Health Authority

Needs assessment methods: Research was carried out by Sheffield Hallam University, with additional evidence from Rockingham Drug Project

Target age groups: 11 and over

Target groups: Users of injectables, opiates; not at school; homeless

Methods and evaluation: The work is done on a one-to-one or small group basis with young drug users, either in person or on the telephone. This is a confidential service which offers advice, support and practical help.

Records are kept by workers on the programme of each client, and feedback is recorded. Monthly reports are written by the team leader.

Drug education for young people

This is an initiative to provide accurate, honest and up-to-date information about drug-related issues in order to enable young people to make healthier, better informed decisions about their drug use.

Contact: Susie Skyes

Tel: 0114 272 9164

Funders: Single Regeneration Budget

Needs assessment methods: The assessment was based on research carried out by Sheffield Hallam University on the place and meaning of drugs in the lives of young people. This was followed by a three-month investigation into services and gaps in services both locally and nationally.

Target age groups: 11 and over

Methods and evaluation: A programme of three workshops is offered to schools and carried out by a team of credible, trained volunteers. Activity-based work is carried out in less formal environments, such as youth groups. This may involve drama, art work, etc. Discussion-based work is sometimes carried out on the streets and at community events such as festivals.

Ongoing monitoring and evaluation systems have been set up in conjunction with the funders. They are based on feedback from all participants, recording of feedback from professionals, and evaluation records kept by volunteers and staff on all activities undertaken. Monthly reports are produced by the team leader.

Safer Dancing Initiative

This aims to reduce drug-related harm in all-night venues through the provision of an information stall, on-hand advice and a first-aid service.

Contact: Anna Christophorou

Tel: 0114 272 9164

Partners: Local Authority Licensing Committee

Funders: Single Regeneration Budget

Needs assessment methods: A survey of 700 clubbers at all-night venues was carried out.

Target age groups: 17 and over

Methods and evaluation: Clubs and sound systems are currently offered a package consisting of one paid worker and three volunteers. They are responsible for providing advice and first aid; this includes a talkdown service and drugs information stall.

The project is evaluated by Rachel Massey, Sheffield University. Due to the nature of the activity, evaluation will predominantly be qualitative.

Youth justice project

The project provides drugs advice, information, one-to-one counselling and education specifically for young people involved with the criminal justice system. It aims to reduce drug-related harm, tackle drugs problems, and reduce drug-related offending.

Contact: Janine Scorthorne

Tel: 0114 272 9164

Partners: Family and community services; Probation Service; South Yorkshire Police; Sheffield Solicitors; Magistrates Court; HM Prison Service

Funders: South Yorkshire Police Authorities; Sheffield Safer Cities

Needs assessment methods: A needs assessment was conducted by managers of family and community services and by the youth justice team.

Target age groups: 11 and over

Target groups: Offenders; young people in trouble with the law

Methods and evaluation: The project provides telephone advice; one-to-one counselling; education workshops; referral for detox and rehab; liaison with all agencies in the criminal justice system; support in court; support on release from prison; and support dealing with family and friends.

Evaluation is by a six-month basic report, but it aims to have an evaluation by an independent organisation at a later date.

SOUTH YORKSHIRE POLICE

50 Windsor Road, Heeley, Sheffield, South Yorkshire S8 8UB

Tel: 0114 282 1209   **Fax:** 0114 282 1208

Contact: Inspector J P W Beresford

Health authority: Sheffield

Main business: Prevention of crime and community safety, in addition to prosecutions

The Lifestyle Project

The object of Lifestyle is to encourage young people aged 9–18 years to work in teams with an adult adviser to improve, where possible, the quality of life for others in the community. Activity takes place during the summer school holidays and teams work on individual projects of their choice. This helps participants to beat boredom, raise self-esteem and avoid becoming involved in crime.

Contact: Inspector J P W Beresford

Tel: 0114 282 1209

Partners: Local Education Authority, Council for Voluntary Service; local business; RailTrack; Rural Action; Remploy; local media; Single Regeneration Budget funded groups in South Yorkshire

Funders: South Yorkshire Police; businesses

Target age groups: 9–18

Target groups: Offenders; black Caribbean; black African; black other; Indian; Pakistani; Bangladeshi; not at school; children in care; parents (carers of children); neighbourhood watch

Methods and evaluation: The Lifestyle Project is run as a competition to encourage young people to spend their spare time constructively during the school summer holidays. Teams of between three and five youngsters register with the police to receive a starter pack, which comprises a free T-shirt and baseball cap, then choose a project to improve the lifestyle of others in their community. In so doing they have fun, beat boredom and avoid crime.

Evaluation is by a resident survey in a selected area; crime statistics analysis; and the user groups

Crucial Crew

The project aims to promote social responsibility and community safety, and to raise drug awareness and safety.

Contact: Inspector J P W Beresford

Tel: 0114 282 1209

Partners: Fire service; Health Authority; ambulance service; British Telecom; community nursing; Victim Support; colleges of further education

Funders: South Yorkshire Police; Local Education Authority

Target age group: 11–16

Target groups: Black Caribbean; black African; black other; Indian; Pakistani; Bangladeshi

Methods: A Crucial Crew centre is formed in each of the metropolitan borough areas, usually in disused schools or other buildings. The police and other agencies join forces to set up approximately 10 scenarios which featured an aspect of danger, from road safety to drugs. Children in groups not exceeding 10 in number visit each scenario and learn the correct way in which to act.

SOUTH YORKSHIRE POLICE CRIME AND COMMUNITY SERVICES

Snig Hill, Sheffield, South Yorkshire S3 8LY

Tel: 0114 252 3493   **Fax:** 0114 252 3421

Contact: Carol Fletcher

Health authority: Sheffield

Other drug services: Community safety; criminal justice; training

Main business: Police training in relation to young people

Drugs education and prevention

The services provide training, resourcing and policy.

Contact: Carol Fletcher

Tel: 0114 252 3493

Partners: Local Education Authority; health voluntary sector

Funder: South Yorkshire Police

Target group: Parents

Evaluation: This is through individual forms.

West Yorkshire

BAC (BLACK AGAINST CRACK)

c/o Youth Reach, Hennymoor House, 7 Manor Row, Bradford, West Yorkshire BD1 4PB

Tel: 01274 720196

Contact: Wayne Allen

Health authority: Bradford

Other drug services: Treatment; training

Peer education

The organisation aims to equip peer educators with essential knowledge skills and experience in order to train/inform their peer groups, and to help build confidence and self-esteem.

Contact: Wayne Allen

Tel: 01274 480805

Partners: Allerton Young People's Project; Bradford Drug Prevention Initiative; Bradford HIV Unit

Funders: Consortium

Target age groups: 11 and over

Target group: Neighbourhoods

Evaluation: This is carried out by the Bradford Drug Prevention Team and peer education staff, and involves external group discussion, an evaluation form, and supervision.

BRADFORD WORKING WOMEN'S PROJECT

11 Hallfield Road, Manningham, Bradford, West Yorkshire BD1 3RP

Tel: 01274 741357

Contact: Carolyn Henham

Health authority: Bradford

Other drug services: Treatment; training; acupuncture

Main business: HIV/sexual health work with women involved in prostitution

Drugs peer education

The project aims: to identify and contact young women who are vulnerable to drug use and prostitution (or already involved); to identify and respond to the needs of young women in relation to drug use; to work with a small group to train as peer educators and to provide support, training and counselling for that group.

Contact: Carolyn Henham

Tel: 01274 741357

Partners: Bradford Social Services (Joint Finance)

Funders: Central Drugs Prevention; West Yorkshire Drug Prevention Team

Target age groups: 11 and over

Target groups: Offenders; women; users of heroin, crack/cocaine; not at school; homeless; children in care

DRUGSWATCH MANAGEMENT COMMITTEE

c/o Police Sergeant Chris Plowman, Central Police Station, The Tyrb, Bradford,
West Yorkshire BD1 1TR

Tel: 01274 376430   **Fax:** 01274 376494   **e-mail:** chris3545@aol.com

Health authority: Bradford

Bradford Drugswatch Drugs Free Premises

This initiative aims to encourage the owners/managers of all entertainment venues in the city centre to take an active role in combating drugs misuse.

Contact: Chris Plowman

Tel: 01274 376430

Partners: Probation; education; pharmaceutical committee; City Centre Manager; magistrates; Health Authority

Funders: Drugswatch Management Committee; West Yorkshire Police

Needs assessment methods: A need for Drugs Free Premises was driven by popular demand – both from the public and the management of venues.

Target age groups: 11 and over

MANNINGHAM DRUG FORUM

2 Duckworth Lane, Bradford, West Yorkshire BD4 0DF

Tel: 01274 488382

Contact: Laila Ahmed

Health authority: Bradford

Drug awareness open day

The aim of the open day is to promote the idea of 'drug awareness' with parents and elders of the Bradford Asian community.

Contact: Laila Ahmed

Tel: 01274 488382

Partner: Manningham Clinic

Needs assessment methods:
A questionnaire was sent out to assess the need for the project.

Target groups: Indian; Pakistani; Bangladeshi; parents; Bradford Asian community

Methods: The day is a drop-in provision for adults. Stalls on offer provide information on drug agency contacts, the effects of drug use, and how to stop smoking.

MILLAN CENTRE

Victor Street, Manningham, Bradford, West Yorkshire BD9 4RA

Tel: 01274 480691

Contact: Pam Hardisty

Health authority: Bradford

Main business: Women's and girls' community centre offering social activities, training, crèche, and girls' groups

Drama project with Asian girls

This project centres on drama-based group work.

Contact: Cath Tearne

Tel: 01274 480691

Partner: West Yorkshire Drug Action Team

Funders: Home Office; Millan Centre

Target age group: 11–16

Target groups: Indian; Pakistani; Bangladeshi; women; neighbourhoods

Evaluation: The project will be evaluated through interviews and questionnaires.

Drugs awareness project

This project aims to inform and empower women and girls to deal with increasing drug use in the area.

Contact: Pam Hardisty

Tel: 01274 480691

Partners: Bridge Project; West Yorkshire Drug Action Team

Funders: West Yorkshire Drug Action Team; Millan Centre

Target groups: Pakistani; women; parents; neighbourhoods

Methods: The project includes the following methods: outreach to schools and door-to-door; workshops; work with parents; alternative strategies; relaxation, etc.; campaigning; signposting to other agencies; and bringing support agencies to the centre support groups.

NO TO NASHA

Central House, Forster Square, Bradford, West Yorkshire BD1 1DJ

Tel: 01274 754489   **Fax:** 01274 740839

Contact: Gurpaul Sandhu

Health authority: Bradford

No to Nasha

The project aims to prevent drug abuse in Asian/Afro-Caribbean communities and other ethnic minorities by providing low-cost, drug-free diversionary activities. It also encourages discussion between young people and their parents about drug issues, so that the existing problems can be dealt with more readily by an informed community.

Contact: Gurpaul Sandhu

Tel: 01274 754489

Partners: Bradford Community Health; NHS Trust; community organisations

Funders: Department of Recreation; Health Authority; Area Regeneration; Drug Action Team

Needs assessment methods: Discussion evenings and seminars were held with parents' groups, young people and representatives from Asian businesses.

Target age groups: 11 and over

Target groups: Black Caribbean; black African; Indian; Pakistani; Bangladeshi; not at school; parents

Methods and evaluation: The campaign features high-profile community events involving debates, music and sporting activities.

Each event is followed by informal discussion and feedback from participants.

ROYDS DRUGS INITIATIVE

Buttershaw Youth Centre, Reevy Road, Buttershaw, Bradford, West Yorkshire BD6 3PU

Tel: 01274 679985

Contact: Ian Roberts

Health authority: Bradford

Development of parent/resident group

The group was formed to give information and support to concerned residents and parents, and to encourage parents and residents to become actively involved in the education and development of young people through planning activity days.

Contact: Emma Marshall

Tel: 01274 788158

Funders: Drug Prevention Team; Crime Reduction Action Group

Target groups: Parents; neighbourhoods; concerned residents

Methods and evaluation: Training days were arranged for residents/parents at the end of which an action plan session was held. Problems and concerns were addressed as well as what action could be taken to tackle these problems and alleviate concerns. Regular fortnightly meetings were arranged. Speakers have since been brought in and the group has planned and helped to run youth activity days. The group is planning more work with young people and would like to design parent help packs.

Evaluation is through discussion at the beginning of each meeting to review aims and progress

Youth activity days

The main aim is to run various workshops for young people around the theme of image (how they see themselves and where they live); to look at positive aspects of their lives; to give them a means of expression; and to look at ways of meeting their needs.

Contact: Emma Marshall

Tel: 01274 788158

Funders: Drug Prevention Initiative; Crime Prevention Action Group

Needs assessment methods:
Questionnaires, surveys and general discussions over a one-year period culminated in a day-long action planning day, where this information was used as a basis to plan future activities.

Target age groups: 11 and over

Methods and evaluation: Activity days are planned around the theme of 'self image'. The days are free and are advertised around the estate. The first day is art and craft-based, followed by a visual arts workshop run by Theatre In the Mill, including dance, drama, creative writing, drawing, photography and the use of camcorders. Over the weekend young people look at their life situation and think about what they like and dislike.

At each of the events evaluation posters are put on the walls and young people are encouraged to write down what they thought of the day and what other activities they would like to do.

Youth empowerment group

This group is being formed to allow older youths (12+) to meet on a regular basis and to take action to improve their life situation, discuss problems and access training. The focus of the activity will be decided by the young people involved.

Contact: Pat Carter

Tel: 01274 674812

Partners: Royds Regeneration Youth Strategy Group; Community Development Team

Funders: Drug Prevention Initiative; Crime Reduction Action Group

Needs assessment methods: A youth worker talked to young people to assess what they needed. The main requirement was a meeting place where they could relax and talk.

Target age groups: 12 and over

Target group: Non-youth club users

Methods: A building on the estate was acquired for community use, with rooms used as youth meeting places. Young people can design, decorate and furnish rooms, and there are plans to turn part of the building into a café – in the hope that young people from the group will run it as an evening meeting place for other youths.

X-PLOSION PROJECT

Youth Reach, Hennymoore House, 7 Manor Row, Bradford, West Yorkshire BD1 4PB

Tel: 01274 720196   **Fax:** 01274 739606

Contact: Emile Peltier

Health authority: Bradford

National tour

The tour involves one-off events in 25 major cities to facilitate a forum for other agencies to distribute material or publicise their drugs initiatives, using music as a medium.

Contact: Emile Peltier

Tel: 01274 720196

Partners: West Yorkshire Drug Prevention Unit; health promotion agencies; police; Social Services

Funders: Drug Prevention Unit; Health Promotion Unit/Service, council recreation; X-Plosion

Needs assessment methods: Pilot venues were evaluated.

Target age groups: 11–18

Methods and evaluation: The tour included: workshops; police workshops; drama workshops; art workshops, music workshops; and a drug agency. A musical event allowed young people to enjoy themselves, thereby creating a friendly and real environment for agencies to provide young people and adults with information.

Each agency evaluates their own effectiveness, and X-Plosion collates these to provide a holistic evaluation.

Recreational/community performances

The aim is to support local events, such as Bradford Festival, the Lord Mayor's Appeal, Heart Smart, and other community events.

Contact: Emile Peltier

Tel: 01274 720196

Partners: Bradford Council; Social Services

Funders: Council projects; X-Plosion fundraising

Target groups: Black Caribbean; Indian; Pakistani; Bangladeshi

Methods and evaluation: Live performance, stalls, art/drama workshops, audience participation, prizes, games, etc. are all part of this activity. Musical equipment and DJs are provided, as well as publicity of the event to users and participants. Other projects/agencies may display their messages (including messages not specifically drugs related, e.g. sex education, homelessness, crime initiatives).

Youth clubs, council staff, participants and X-plosion staff evaluate their own effectiveness. Questionnaires are also provided at every venue, which help to evaluate the general public opinion, preferences, complaints and desires. This is made available to other agencies.

ASIAN DRUGS PROJECT (HALIFAX)

31 St Johns Lane, Halifax, West Yorkshire HX1 2QQ

Tel: 01422 361111   **Fax:** 01422 346092

Contact: Christine Clavering

Health authority: Calderdale and Kirklees

Other drug services: Treatment; community safety

Main business: Helping Asian drug users with issues around drugs

Alternative activities

This initiative is aimed at helping Asians who are at risk of being involved with drugs to gain knowledge, formulate attitudes, and share ideas around drugs and drug use.

Contact: Nadeeem Mirza

Tel: 01422 361111

Funder: West Yorkshire Drug Prevention Team

Target groups: Asians; neighbourhoods

Methods and evaluation: Group discussions around drug use take place within the Asian community: how drugs affect the body both long and short term; how drugs have destroyed many Asian families; where to get help. Aim to challenge attitudes.

Evaluation is through before-and-after questionnaires, and discussions on various drugs.

CALDERDALE HEALTH PROMOTION UNIT

Health Promotion Centre, 47 Crown Street, Halifax, West Yorkshire HX1 1JB

Tel: 01422 366733

Contact: Tony Pye

Health authority: Calderdale and Kirklees

Other drug services: Treatment; needle exchange

Outreach and support

The aim of this work is to support/advise and target young people who are using substances through outreach activities with parents, youth and community staff.

Contact: Karen Brooke

Tel: 01422 361111

Partner: Dashline – Street Agency

Funders: Health Authority; Health Promotion Unit/Service

Needs assessment methods: Discussions with professionals highlighted the gaps in the provision of services for young people.

Target age groups: 11 and over

Target groups: Parents; disadvantaged

Methods: Active, experimental, pairs, and group discussions, and use of games, etc. are all employed in the work.

COMMUNITY EDUCATION SERVICE – CALDERDALE METROPOLITAN BOROUGH COUNCIL

Education Department, Northgate House, Northgate, Halifax, West Yorkshire HX1 1UN

Tel: 01422 392528   **Fax:** 01422 392515

Contacts: Dave Cooper, Patrick Ambrose

Health authority: Calderdale and Kirklees

Main business: Community education

Young People, Drugs and Decisions

The aim of this initiative was to provide programmes which raised awareness and reduced harm, through youth arts, in selected youth organisations in the borough. The project finished in February 1996.

Contact: Patrick Ambrose

Tel: 01422 351802

Partners: Calderdale and Kirklees Health Authority; Calderdale Health Promotion Unit/Service

Funders: Calderdale and Kirklees Health Authority; Calderdale Metropolitan Borough Council Community Education Service; National Health Service

Methods and evaluation: A number of youth arts workers were introduced to a series of youth clubs in order to develop young people's ideas around drugs education. Accurate information and group discussions were also used.

Evaluation was by feedback sheets; group discussions; individual interviews; and observation.

DASHLINE

31 St John's Lane, Halifax, West Yorkshire HX1 2QQ

Tel: 01422 361111   **Fax:** 01422 346092

Contact: Karen Brooke

Health authority: Calderdale and Kirklees

Other drug services: Treatment; training

Peer Education Project – Ovender

The aim of the project is to work with young people and examine issues around drug use, and to help young people to produce a peer education package.

Contact: Karen Brooke

Tel: 01422 361111

Partners: GARTA; Youth Empowerment Project – Ovenders

Target age groups: 11–18

Target groups: Neighbourhoods

Methods: Peer education methods take place during five sessions in one weekend.

Youth forum – Brighouse and Rastrick area

The aim of the forum is to establish a group of young people who will meet regularly and discuss the best way to address local substance use, the problems of young people, development of strategies regarding substance use with workers, and the distribution of small grants to fund young people's own initiatives regarding substance use.

Contact: Karen Brooke

Tel: 01422 361111

Partner: Community education youth service

Funder: Health Authority

Target age groups: 11–21

Target group: Neighbourhoods

Methods: Young people are encouraged to manage their own grant process for substance use prevention work, and to establish the priorities and criteria for grants. In time the group may serve as a general consultancy group for professional workers.

DASHLINE – PONTEFRACT AND DISTRICT DRUG SOLVENT HELPLINE

Southmoor House, Southmoor Road, Hemsworth, Pontefract, West Yorkshire WF9 HSQ

Tel: 01977 617045   **Fax:** 01977 617045

Contact: John Bates

Health authority: Wakefield

Other drug services: Treatment; community safety; training

Outreach work

The work involves presentations, client contact, schools, licensed premises and youth clubs.

Contact: John Bates

Tel: 01977 617045

Funders: National Lottery Charities Board; Single Regeneration Budget; Comic Relief; Wakefield Health Authority

Target groups: Not at school; children in care; parents; neighbourhoods.

UNIT 51

36–38 Portland Street, Huddersfield, West Yorkshire HO1 5PL

Tel: 01484 510826   **Fax:** 01484 548701   **e-mail:** Unit51@geo1.poptel.org.uk

Contact: Colin Wisely

Health authority: Calerdale and Kirklees

Other drug services: Treatment; community safety; criminal justice; training; outreach; structured day programmes

Young people's early intervention work

Early intervention is achieved by providing outreach in pubs and clubs, advice and information, parent/family work, counselling and support, training, research, licence training, and youth drug forums.

Contact: Carole Dennet

Tel: 01484 510826

Funders: West Yorkshire Drug Prevention Team; Health Authority

Target age groups: 11–21

Target groups: Offenders; black Caribbean; black African; black other; parents; rural communities

Evaluation: West Yorkshire Drug Prevention Team evaluates the project.

AXIS

PO Box XG79, Leeds, West Yorkshire LS14 2XU

Tel: 0113 222 5507   **Fax:** 0113 222 5362   **e-mail:** cic@easynet.co.uk

Contact: Karen Knapton

Health authority: Leeds

Other drug services: Training

Lifestyle

Teams of up to five young people (with an adult adviser) design and implement projects over the summer holidays that benefit their community. Young people receive information on drugs and relevant services as well as gaining improving skills. The project finished in October 1996, and started again in the summer of 1997.

Contact: Karen Knapton

Tel: 0113 222 5507

Partners: West Yorkshire Police, Killingbeck; Leeds Local Education Authority; various schools

Funders: Children in Crisis; police, Yorkshire Electricity; West Yorkshire Drug Prevention Team

Target age groups: 11–18

Target groups: Not at school

Methods and evaluation: Young people are contacted through schools, the youth service, education welfare, etc. They form teams, and identify a project they can do over the summer holidays. As part of the package, young people are given information on drugs.

Teams are asked to keep a log book, and those teams judged to have put in the most effort and to have had a major effect on their community are positively rewarded. Young people are given the option to link in with existing accreditation schemes, e.g. Record Achievement, Duke of Edinburgh Award, and training qualifications.

Outdoor Pursuits Climbing Project

Axis aims to run a rolling programme of outdoor activities with young people in East Leeds – the first activity being climbing.

Contact: Karen Knapton

Tel: 0113 222 5507

Partners: Leeds youth and community services; Killingbeck Police Division (Leeds)

Funders: Children in Crisis; Leeds youth and community services; police

Target age group: 11–16

Target groups: Neighbourhoods; rural communities

Methods: Each group of young people attends a 12-week programme, which includes tuition on a climbing wall and training in map reading, knots, etc. This culminates in a short stay at a hostel in the Dales. The young people learn basic climbing skills, team work and planning skills for the trip to the hostel, including budgeting for food, etc. Those completing the course then attend a practical assessment which, if they pass, allows them to continue the activity without direct supervision at a local climbing wall.

AZUKA PROJECT

20b Grange Terrace, Chapeltown, Leeds, LS7 4EF

Tel: 0113 237 4707

Contact: Joseph Gatewood

Health authority: Leeds

Other drug services: Treatment; criminal justice; training; counselling; assessment; acupuncture; advocacy

Drug education/training

The aim is: to increase knowledge about drugs and dispel myths; to provide accurate information about drug use and its risks; and to develop harm reduction skills regarding safer drug use.

Contact: Joseph Gatewood

Tel: 0113 237 4707

Needs assessment methods: Discussions with staff and pupils; and questionnaires were completed to assess the need for this project.

Target age groups: 11 and over

Target groups: Black Caribbean; black African; black other; Indian; Pakistani; Bangladeshi; not at school; homeless; parents

Evaluation: Questionnaires revealed that young people felt that drug education should be accessible to other young people within the schooling system.

HAKIM YOUTH FORUM

10 Reginald Mount, Chapeltown, Leeds, West Yorkshire LS7 3HN

Tel: 01973 724276

Contact: Nadeem Javeed

Health authority: Leeds

Drug Stop!

The project aims to increase awareness of drug abuse, pinpoint vices, and give solutions through training. It also works to curb drugs at a young age, through plays at schools and colleges.

Contact: Nadeem Javeed

Tel: 01973 724276

Funders: Self-funding

Target groups: Offenders; not at school; homeless; children in care; parents; community groups

Methods and evaluation: The following activities are used: plays staged at schools; seminars on drug misuse; liaison with police and community elders; the Internet; and trips to residentials in Wales and France.

Evaluation takes the form of minute taking, questionnaires, feedback, and public opinion.

HEALTH EDUCATION

Burton Road Centre, Burton Avenue, Leeds, West Yorkshire LS11 5EA

Tel: 0133 271 9197   **Fax:** 0113 277 6339

Contact: Maggie Jackson

Health authority: Leeds

Other drug services: Training

Main business: Health education, supporting youth work

City centre detached substance use team

Detached youth workers meet young people on the street in the city centre, offer information and support, and assist young people with referrals to treatment agencies.

Contact: Maggie Jackson

Tel: 0133 271 9197

Partners: Young People's Information Centre

Funders: Leeds City Council

Needs assessment methods: A pilot project identified a number of young people involved in substance use in the locality. It also recorded concerns/complaints from local shopkeepers, police, etc.

Target age groups: 11 and over

Target groups: Users of solvents; neighbourhoods

Methods: Detached youth workers have developed positive relationships with growing numbers of young people who congregate in the city centre and have drug habits in common. Workers are always at particular contact points at certain times in the week. Most of the work is one-to-one, although initially a group of young people took part in making a video. Workers now offer information on a range of issues (benefits, relationships) as well as substance use. They help to make referrals to treatment agencies and will accompany young people to the appointments.

Health education youth and community

This is a support team for area-specific youth workers in their planning, resourcing and delivery of health education (including drug prevention) programmes. It also works with parents/community groups, and has developed an HIV peer-led project, which includes substance use and harm minimisation.

Contact: Maggie Jackson

Tel: 0133 271 9197

Partners: Health Authority

Funders: Leeds City Council; Health Authority

Needs assessment methods: A survey of the area youth work teams, in October 1990, identified a need.

Target age groups: 11 and over

Target groups: Parents; community groups

LEEDS HEALTH PROMOTION SERVICE (LHPS)

St Mary's Hospital, Greenhill Road, Armley, Leeds, West Yorkshire LS12 3QE

Tel: 0113 279 0121   **Fax:** 0113 231 0185

Contact: Judith Knapton

Health authority: Leeds

Other drug services: Training

Family of Schools Drugs Initiative

The initiative aims to provide a co-ordinated and consistent drugs education programme as part of a wider health education framework involving two families of schools within Leeds, and to increase the links between the schools and local communities.

Contact: Judith Knapton

Tel: 0113 279 0121

Partners: Leeds Local Education Authority; City Council Youth and Community; AXIS (Children in Crisis); Bramley and Rodley Community Action; West Yorkshire Drug Prevention Team

Funders: West Yorkshire Drug Prevention Team; Steering Group members

Needs assessment methods: Discussions with schools and relevant agencies within Leeds revealed that drug education was patchy, and that its links with communities varied.

Target groups: Schools and communities

Methods and evaluation: The West Yorkshire Drug Prevention Team has commissioned the Research and Services Development Centre to carry out baseline research of the current provision. This information will then be disseminated through workshops with each 'family' to develop a programme specific to each area. The content and methods of delivery will be decided by each area.

West Yorkshire Drug Prevention Team has commisioned an independent researcher, Dr Susan Harris, to evaluate the process and outcome.

Jewish Community Drug Awareness Programme

This programme aims to raise awareness of substance use issues in the community.

Contacts: Judith Knapton, Diane Tilman

Tel: 0113 279 0121

Partners: Schools; police

Funder: Leeds Jewish community

Needs assessment methods: Informal discussions within the community were carried out by the community to assess the need to raise awareness.

Target groups: Parents

Methods: The community has run a series of awareness-raising sessions from which ideas for other initiatives/events have developed.

Resources for Asian Communities

This is an initiative to develop resources for use within Asian communities.

Contact: Judith Knapton

Tel: 0113 279 0121

Partner: Black Communities AIDS Team (BCAT)

Funder: Leeds Health Promotion Unit/Service

Needs assessment methods: There was an assessment of resources locally and nationally as well as discussions with Asian workers in Leeds.

Target age groups: 11–18

Target groups: Black Caribbean; black African; black other

Methods: Discussions were held with Asian workers, followed by work with focus groups of young Asians to establish what kind of resources would be most useful. The resources were then developed with young Asians, followed by piloting the resources, production and dissemination.

A follow-up evaluation was made.

TURNING POINT – LEEDS YOUNG PEOPLE

60 Upper Basinghall Street, Leeds, West Yorkshire LS1 5HR

Tel: 0113 243 3552

Contact: Caroline Smith

Health authority: Leeds

Intervention service

This is a confidential and non-judgemental early intervention service for young substance users in Leeds at risk of harm from such use. It aims: to provide confidential advice, information, support and counselling to young people, to minimise substance-related harm; and to involve young people in the shaping, evaluation and delivery of the service.

Contact: Caroline Smith

Tel: 0113 243 3552

Funder: Health Authority

Needs assessment methods: Resource and Service Development Centre research included the following: a questionnaire to young people identifying areas of need (1996); a mapping exercise (1995); Health Promotion survey (1994); and Resource and Service Development Centre survey of schools (1995).

Target age groups: 11 and over

Methods and evaluation: The service aims to be flexible, and to be able to respond to young people's needs. It offers a telephone advice line, counselling and support on a one-to-one basis. There are short drug and alcohol awareness packages available, and support is offered to those working with young people who use substances. Information and harm minimisation materials will be developed, and a model of peer education devised.

Evaluation is in the form of questionnaires, audit, appraisal, and supervision.

WEST LEEDS DRUG PROJECT

Bramley Community Centre, Waterloo Lane, Leeds, West Yorkshire LS13 2JB

Tel: 0113 236 1713

Contact: Clair Dowgill

Health authority: Leeds

Other drug services: Treatment; community safety; criminal justice; training; information and support on non-drug-related issues.

Substance Use/Misuse Project (SUP)

The project works with young people around all drug issues.

Contact: Sonia Sharp

Tel: 0113 236 1713

Partner: West Leeds Works Exchange

Funders: Comic Relief; Safer Cities

Needs assessment methods: A need was identified through work carried out by police, the social services, youth provision and schools in the area.

Target age groups: 11 and over

Target groups: Offenders; not at school; homeless; children in care; parents; neighbourhoods; community groups

Methods and evaluation: SUP goes into any environment where young people will be. It uses a variety of media to raise awareness: videos, leaflets, games, questionaires, one-to-one, and group discussion.

Evaluation is through: three-monthly reports to funders to secure continuing funding; questionnaires and face-to-face discussion with clients/groups; school feedback; regular team meetings; and supervision.

ARCADE (A RURAL COMMUNITY APPROACH TO DRUG EDUCATION)

Netherton Village Hall, 330–2 Meltham Road, Netherton, West Yorkshire HD4 7EX

Tel: 01484 667705   **Fax:** 01484 666419

Contact: Kate Gimblett

Health authority: Calderdale and Kirklees

Community development and drug education

Activities centre on drug education with local adults to raise awareness; community arts with young people; stimulating interest in young people; and creating a community forum for ongoing contact between young people and adults.

Contact: Peter Hardy

Tel: 01484 667705

Funders: Drug Prevention; Rural Development; Health Authority

Target age groups: 11–21

Target groups: Parents; neighbourhoods; community groups; rural communities

Community development services

Activities involve youth work and drug education.

Contact: Theresa Dyson

Tel: 01484 667705

Needs assessment methods: A drug questionnaire was distributed.

Target age groups: 11–21

Target groups: Rural communities

Methods and evaluation: The service employs the following methods: flipcharts describing what a drug is; what effects drugs have; classifications of drugs; legal facts on drugs; leaflets available at all times in youth club on drugs; and Lifeline material for young people in the club who have used illegal drugs such as Ecstasy, LSD and amphetamines.

Evaluation is by questionnaires to participants.

GASPED (GROUP AWARENESS AND SUPPORT FOR PARENTS ENCOUNTERING DRUGS)

182 Kingsway, Ossett, West Yorkshire WF5 8DW

Tel: 01924 265678

Contact: Kristine Smith

Health authority: Wakefield

Other drug services: Help and support to parents/families of drug users; helpline contact; fortnightly meetings for parents

GASPED

The group's main aim is to offer help, advice, information and support to parents/families of drug users through group therapy and to provide education on drugs awareness and drug-related problems. A helpline is also available.

Contact: Kristine Smith

Tel: 01924 275591

Funders: Self-funded; charities

Target groups: Parents

Methods: The group offers a helpline for advice, and for those who need someone to listen to their problems (information leaflets and booklets can be posted out). Parents are encouraged to attend group meetings to meet others with similar problems. The meetings are structured to educate and to make participants more aware of drugs and related problems, e.g. treatments, harm reduction, laws, crime, etc. Speakers are invited for special talks, and parents are encouraged to talk openly and explore their own attitudes, opinions and feelings while receiving support. A confidentiality policy is in operation.

OP2

The Brickhouse, Prospect Road, Ossett, Wakefield, West Yorkshire WF5 8AE

Tel: 01924 267244   **Fax:** 01924 267244

Contact: Carol Mennell

Health authority: Wakefield

Other drug services: Training

Main business: Empowering young people; offering the opportunity for support, challenge and achievement.

OP2

The project aims: to empower young people so that they can address the issue of drug prevention and pass on their knowledge to other young people; to increase access for young people to up-to-date information; to make a video by young people; and to provide peer education and a drop-in centre.

Contact: Carol Mennell

Tel: 01924 267244

Funders: West Yorkshire Drug Prevention Team; Wakefield Youth Service

Target age groups: 11–18

Methods: The project offers the following: developing workshops and discussion groups leading to peer education training; establishing skills and knowledge in the production of a video; delivering drugs prevention awareness to others through peer education and a video; providing access to information through a drop-in service.

Appendix 1

Sources of funding

National agencies that fund drug-related projects or services were identified by means of:

- the mapping project;
- SCODA files;
- directories such as *A guide to the major trusts 1995–96 edition*, volume 1:
  The top 300 trusts – published by the Directory of Social Change, 1995.

Each agency was contacted to check its funding criteria. Then access information was compiled, based on literature produced by the agency.

Several national sources of funding for drug education and prevention are detailed on the following pages.

As drug education and prevention activity often attracts local financial support, funding opportunities are also available through local drug forums and networks.

Sources of funding for drug education and prevention

Funding source	Area of interest	Who can apply?	Level of funding	For further information
The Baring Foundation	The Baring Foundation is concerned with: • community regeneration • the changing nature of work • collaborative and inter-disciplinary activity. The specific grants programme aims to strengthen the voluntary sector by supporting initiatives that: • enhance the skills and effectiveness of small or community organisations; • assist two or more charities to consider or implement new joint structures, other forms of formal collaboration, or mergers.	Applications are encouraged from voluntary organisations that work in: • the arts; • education; • environment and conservation; • health and social welfare. Preference is likely to be given to proposals that make links between two or more of these categories. Applications must be from: • local projects in London, Merseyside and the North-East of England (applications from local projects in other areas will not be considered); • national voluntary organisations (including organisations that service only one country within the UK as well as UK-wide organisations); • UK charities with partners in developing countries.	£2000–£10,000	The Baring Foundation 60 London Wall London EC2M 5TQ Tel: 0171 767 1000
Drugs Challenge Fund (Central Drugs Co-ordination Unit)	Challenge funding supports local partnerships through a combination of government support and commitment from the private sector. The funding is competitive, not routinely distributed. It was designed to support initiatives that: • delivered specific outcomes by 31 March against at least two of the three objectives of the Statement of Purpose in *Tackling drugs together* (increasing community safety; reducing acceptability and availability of drugs to young people; reducing health risks of drug misuse); • demonstrate effective local partnerships, including evidence of a clear commitment from the private sector to finance at least a third of the total cost of the proposed initiative; • were capable of completion by 31 March or of being sustained through resources apart from this fund; • build on good practice and represent value for money; • include arrangements for the evaluation of each project by the CDCU.	Drug Action Teams operating in England.	£2 million for 1996/7 only. This comes from a partnership comprising the Treasury, Home Office, Department of Health, and Department for Education and Employment. At least a third of the total cost of the proposed initiative must be committed by the private sector. Options for further partnership work through Challenge funding will be considered at the end of 1996. If it is successful, it may be extended over a longer timespan.	CDCU Room 67D/4 Government Offices Great George Street London SW1P 3AL Tel: 0171 270 5776 Fax: 0171 270 5857

Funding source	Area of interest	Who can apply?	Level of funding	For further information
Esmée Fairbairn Charitable Trust NB The following information is based on the trust's policies for 1995–6 and may be subject to change or revision in 1997.	The trust makes general grants under five specific categories: • arts and heritage; • education; • environment; • social and economic research; • social welfare. The trust's policy with regard to social welfare is that it 'prefers prevention to palliatives', and both young people and substance abuse are listed as priority fields.	Voluntary organisations that deal with issues within the five categories identified.	More than £10 million: over 3000 applications are received each year. Grants range from £250 to £250,000. There is no established precedent for awarding grants up to a specific percentage of the cost of a project. Grants may be awarded for one year, or phased.	Judith Dunworth Secretary The Esmée Fairbairn Charitable Trust 1 Birdcage Walk London SW1H 9JJ Tel: 0171 227 5400 Fax: 0171 233 0421
	The trust also operates a small grants scheme, including one for voluntary sector drug services. The scheme provides support for: • targeting difficult to reach groups; • facilitating user involvement; • providing publicity or educational material not covered in other budgets; • direct service provision (one-off capital support).	Voluntary drug services in the UK; new services and projects, and those using volunteers, have priority.	£50,000: grants of up to £5000 each were awarded in 1996.	
Department for Education and Employment (DfEE) Grants for Education Support and Training (GEST) 1997–8	Drug Prevention and Schools (grant no. 8) assists primary and secondary schools to deliver effective drug education and to manage drug-related incidents on school premises. The grant can be spent on the direct costs of programmes, including: • training teachers; • developing materials and hiring speakers; • raising the awareness of school governors and parents; • promoting effective inter-agency working.	All local education authorities, subject to satisfactory bids. Priority is given to projects and activities which address: • evidence of acute need; • evidence of direct or prospective benefit to schools; • the quality of training and/or materials; • the extent of involvement of schools in planning and undertaking projects.	Approximately £6 million. Most grants for 1997–8 are expected to be between £25,000 and £100,000, and to be targeted at areas of demonstrably greater need.	Richard Urmston Health Education Team Preparation for Adulthood Division DfEE Sanctuary Buildings Great Smith Street London SW1P 3BT Tel: 0171 925 6216 Fax: 0171 925 6988
	Youth service (grant no. 11) supports youth and community workers in the delivery of (in order of priority): • programmes of drug education and prevention; • programmes of crime prevention arising directly from the evaluation of the Youth Action Scheme; • general youth work training, including part-time staff and volunteer-focused programmes. Bids should reflect this order of priority. Expenditure on the first two objectives will focus mainly on salaries of project workers and support staff; transport, premises and equipment may exceptionally be considered, as may salaries of trainers and curriculum materials. Expenditure on the third objective can include the salaries of trainers and curriculum materials.	All LEAs.	Expenditure in 1997–8 is likely to be lower than in 1996–7, which was £1.1 million. Allocations are based on estimates of young people aged 13–19 in each authority, and subject to each authority receiving a minimum allocation of £5000.	Frances Rogers National Youth Agency and Youth Work Training Team Youth Service and Preparation for Adulthood Division DfEE Tel: 0171 925 5265 Fax: 0171 925 6954

Funding source	Area of interest	Who can apply?	Level of funding	For further information
National Lottery Charities Board (NLCB)	Potentially, all three of the next NLCB rounds: New Opportunities and Choices (in skills, training, education and self-help): Improving People's Living Environment; and Community Involvement.	Registered charities, unregistered charities, and benevolent or philanthropic groups throughout the UK. Small and locally based groups are particularly encouraged to apply. Applications can be for one, two or three-year funding; partial or sole funding; capital costs; revenue costs, including core costs; matching funds for European Structural Funds (ESF) or European Union grants.	In the 1996 funding round on young people, 26 projects with a drugs element received just under £3 million, out of a total of £159 million for 2229 projects.	NLCB Head Office St Vincent House 30 Orange Street London WC2H 7HH Tel: 0171 747 5299 Fax: 0171 747 5214 Minicom: 0171 747 5374 Application Forms: 0345 919191 (Minicom: 0345 556656)
Single Regeneration Budget (SRB) Challenge Fund	The SRB, introduced in April 1994, replaced individual programmes of the Department of Education and the Department of Employment (now DfEE), the Department of Trade and Industry (DTI), and the Home Office. It contributes to sustainable regeneration and economic competitiveness by supporting broad projects run by local partnerships that complement main programmes in a way that meets local needs and priorities. Physical, economic and social regeneration are the objectives of SRB Challenge funded work. SRB literature states that bids may complement or relate to the government's White Paper on drugs. The SRB Challenge Fund supports initiatives which build on good practice and existing initiatives, represent value for money and meet one or more of the following objectives: • to enhance the employment prospects, education and skills of local people; • to encourage sustainable economic growth and wealth creation by improving the competitiveness of the local economy; • protect and improve the environment and infrastructure; • improve housing and housing conditions for local people; • promote initiatives of benefit to minority ethnic groups; • tackle crime and improve community safety; • enhance the quality of life and capacity to contribute to local regeneration of local people.	Bids must be supported by partnerships representing all those with a key interest. The structure of partnerships will reflect the content of the bid and characteristics of the target area or groups. One of the partners, normally a local authority or Training and Enterprise Council (TEC), will lead the bid. In cases where the local authority or the TEC does not have the lead role, it will nonetheless normally be expected to be partner in any bid related to its areas of responsibility.	For Round 3 (April 1997 to March 1999), about £200 million, with £50 million of this available in 1997/8.	Regional government office. Details are available from: Government Office for London 7th Floor Riverwalk House 157–161 Millbank London SW1P 4RT Tel: 0171 217 3062

Appendix 2

Documentation

Government strategy documents and key circulars

Advisory Council on the Misuse of Drugs (1984) *Prevention*. HMSO, London.

Advisory Council on the Misuse of Drugs (1990) *Problem drug use: a review of training*. HMSO, London.

Advisory Council on the Misuse of Drugs (1993) *Drug education in schools: the need for new impetus*. HMSO, London.

Department for Education (1995) *Drug prevention and schools.* Circular number 4/95.

Department for Education and the School Curriculum and Assessment Authority (1995) *Drug education: curriculum guidance for schools*. SCAA, London.

Department of Health (1996) *The task force to review services for drug misusers: report of an independent review of drug treatment services in England*. HMSO, London.

Health Advisory Service (1996) *Children and young people, substance misuse services, the substance of young needs*. HMSO, London.

Office for Standards in Education (1997) *The contribution of youth services to drug education.* HMSO, London.

Office for Standards in Education (1997) *Drug education in schools*. HMSO, London.

Tackling drugs together – a strategy for England 1995–98 (1995). HMSO, London.

Directories of services

National

Alcohol services directory (1995). Alcohol Concern, London.
Tel: 0171 928 7377

Drug problems: where to get help (1992). SCODA, London (this edition out of print).
National listing of agencies offering help, advice and treatment for drug users, their families and friends. It gives information on the services provided by each agency as well as details of residential services, and is comprehensively indexed. New updated edition will be available towards the end of 1997. Updates are available to anyone who already has the 1992 edition.
Tel: 0171 928 9500

Local

Guide to services in Greater Manchester (1996). TACADE/Drugs Prevention Initiative.

Directory of drug training in Greater Manchester (1997). TACADE/Drugs Prevention Initiative.

Drugs and alcohol in Lewisham, directory of services (1996). Lewisham Social Services.

Drug and substance misuse problems? A guide to services in Wandsworth, Lambeth, Southwark, Lewisham and Greenwich (1996). South London Drugs Prevention Team.

Many other local agencies have produced or are producing directories of services in their area. Contact your local DAT or health authority for information.

Appendix 3

Drug Education and Prevention Mapping Project Sample Questionnaire

The Standing Conference on Drug Abuse is undertaking a project to map the range of **drug education and prevention activity** directed at **young people** in England. It is being funded by the Department of Health/Health Education Authority as part of the Government's Tackling Drugs Together strategy.

We are mapping activities provided in the community in different locations including on the streets, in youth centres and others. They may be provided by a single specialist agency, or by partnerships of different agencies. We are **not** mapping drug prevention and education activities that are part of the curriculum, but those that take place in schools with young people are relevant if extra-curricular.

The information gathered will be used as an entry in a **handbook of drug education and prevention**. This will be systematically indexed and will provide an accessible resource for the drug education and prevention community and others. It will provide publicity for projects, support networking, and facilitate the sharing of knowledge about activities, methods, evaluation, funding and other issues. The handbook will also describe the role of agencies which are involved in drug prevention and education but do not necessarily deliver activities themselves, and will steer the reader towards appropriate sources where local, regional and national information can be found.

The accompanying questionnaire is designed to gather information for **a profile of activities** and to help us identify suitable case studies. What follows is a list of criteria which activities need to fulfil to be included in the project.

Criteria

- We wish to include activities whose **aims** are amongst the following:
  - to prevent young people from starting to use drugs;
  - to encourage young people who use drugs to stop using drugs;
  - to minimise harm to those young people who are using drugs.

- Only activities that have taken place in the last six months or will take place in the next six months (i.e. from November 1995 to October 1996) will be included.

- The directory will **exclude** any activity which focuses on:
  - the training and development of staff which assists them to provide drug education and prevention;
  - the care, treatment and rehabilitation of young people who have developed **dependency** on drugs, harmful patterns of substance misuse or disorders in which substance misuse plays a role;
  - community safety and enforcement;
  - curriculum drug education.

Exclusions are covered by other work (including directories) that SCODA and others have published or are undertaking.

If you have any queries about filling in the questionnaire or about the project as a whole, please contact Sarah Waterton or Stephen Taylor at:

Standing Conference on Drug Abuse
32–36 Loman Street
London SE1 0EE
Tel: 0171 928 9500

A. YOUR ORGANISATION'S DETAILS

Please complete this front sheet, section A, for your organisation. Write or type your answer in block capitals or circle YES or NO for each question as appropriate.

1. Name of organisation/project providing drug education and prevention:
   (please write in full with abbreviation in brackets if applicable)

   ....

2. Name of managing or parent organisation (if applicable)

   ....

3. Your postal address ....

   ....

4. Postcode ....

5. Telephone ....

6. Fax ....

7. E-mail address ....

8. Your name..

9. Contact name ....
   (someone able to answer questions about the organisation and its activities for the forseeable future)

10. County/Borough name ....

11. Health Authority area ....

12. Drug Action Team (DAT) Area ....

13. Does your organisation provide other drug services *in addition* to drug education and prevention?
    (if no please go to question 15) .... **YES/NO**

14. Which of the following categories do these services fall into?
    a. treatment and care of drug users .... **YES/NO**
    b. community safety... **YES/NO**
    c. criminal justice .... **YES/NO**
    d. training and development of staff .... **YES/NO**
    e. other .... **YES/NO**
    Please describe briefly ....

15. Is drug work the main business of your organisation?............................... **YES/NO**
    (if yes go to section B)

16. What is the main business of your organisation? ....

    ....

B. *YOUR ACTIVITIES*

Please complete a separate section B for as many different activities as you are running. To facilitate this 3 copies are provided, but please photocopy and fill out more if you are running more than 3 activities which fit the following criteria:

The activity's aims include:

- preventing young people from starting to use drugs;

- encouraging young people who use drugs to stop using drugs;

- minimising harm to those young people who are using drugs.

To be included in the directory the activity needs to have taken place in the last six months or will take place in the next six months (i.e. **from November 1995 to October 1996**).

1. Activity name or a descriptive name ....
    ....

2. Briefly describe the main aim, focus and work of the activity ....
    ....
    ....
    ....

3. Contact name for the activity ....

4. Telephone no. (if different to A5) ....

5. Where does the activity take place?
    a. In schools, colleges, or other formal educational settings .... **YES/NO**
    b   In youth centres, scout huts or other informal educational/recreational settings .... **YES/NO**
    c. On the streets, in parks or other outdoor settings .... **YES/NO**
    d. From a bus or other mobile venue .... **YES/NO**
    e. In pubs or clubs or other commercial recreational venues .... **YES/NO**
    f. In community centres, on estates or in other community settings .... **YES/NO**
    g. Other .... **YES/NO**
    Please give details ....
    ....

6. How many full-time equivalent paid staff work on the activity? ....

7. How many full-time equivalent volunteer staff work on the activity? ....

8. When did the activity start? **Day**   **Month**   **Year**

9. When did/will the activity finish? Either: **Day**   **Month**   **Year**   /or: **ONGOING**

10. How many people has the activity reached and/or how many does it expect to reach between November 1995 and October 1996?

....

11. If the activity is being run in partnership with any other agencies or groups please give their details:

....

....

....

12. Who funds the activity:

    a. major/core funder ....

        ....

    b. secondary funder/supporters ....

        ....

13. Was a needs assessment exercise completed before or during the setting up of the activity?
.... **YES/NO**
(if no go to question 15)

14. What methods were used for the needs assessment and what results were found? ....

    ....

    ....

15. Is the activity *specifically* aimed at reaching one or more of the target groups below?

    a. offenders .... **YES/NO**

    b. ethnic minority groups .... **YES/NO**   if yes, which? ....

    c. specific age groups .... **YES/NO**   if yes, which age group(s)? ....

    d. one gender....................................... **YES/NO**   if yes, which? ....

    e. users of specific drugs .... **YES/NO**   if yes, which? ....

    f.   school excludees/non attenders ...... **YES/NO**

    g. homeless young people .... **YES/NO**

    h. children in care................................ **YES/NO**

    i.   parents/relatives .... **YES/NO**   if yes, specify ....

    j.   particular neighbourhoods................ **YES/NO**

    k. community/tenants groups............... **YES/NO**   if yes, specify ....

    l.   rural communities............................ **YES/NO**

    m. other.. **YES/NO**   if yes, specify ....

16. What methods of drug education and prevention does the activity use?
    a.   educating about drugs and drug use .... **YES/NO**
    b.   peer education .... **YES/NO**
    c.   information and advice provision, e.g. written, telephone, face-to-face .... **YES/NO**
    d.   information development e.g. writing leaflets, designing posters .... **YES/NO**
    e.   practical or social skills learning & development .... **YES/NO**
    f.   art, photography, multimedia .... **YES/NO**
    g.   music, radio, DJ-ing .... **YES/NO**
    h.   sport or other physical activity .... **YES/NO**
    i.   theatre, video, TV .... **YES/NO**
    j.   providing a social centre or place to meet .... **YES/NO**
    k.   community development .... **YES/NO**
    l.   providing funding/expertise/support to others .... **YES/NO**
    m. other .... **YES/NO**

17. Please describe in detail the methods used *(attach an additional sheet if you need more space)*
    ....
    ....
    ....
    ....
    ....
    ....
    ....

18. Has the activity been evaluated?... **YES/NO**
    (if no go to question 21)

19. By whom was it evaluated?
    a.   the participants .... **YES/NO**
    b.   the staff/volunteers... **YES/NO**
    c.   an independent organisation/person.. **YES/NO**
    e.   funder/managing/commissioning body .... **YES/NO**
    f.   other .... **YES/NO**
    Please give details ....
    ....

20. What methods were used for the evaluation and what results were found? ....

....

....

....

....

....

21. If there is any thing else you would like to add about your activity, please write it in the space below

....

....

....

22. What additional information and support (excluding funding!) would be helpful to you in delivering this activity?

....

....

23. Have you any written information relating to your activity, e.g. publicity material, research or evaluation reports? .... **YES/NO**

If YES, and you are able to send us a copy, please send it separately to Sarah Waterton using our freepost address:

Standing Conference on Drug Abuse, FREEPOST LON7663, LONDON, SE1 0YW

If it is in a published book/magazine/journal, please give the reference and any other relevant details

....

....

**Thank you very much indeed for taking
the time to complete this questionnaire.**

**Please return your completed copy in the enclosed
reply-paid envelope by *Friday 14th June*.**

Index of Organisations and Activities by County and Town

Index of Organisations and Activities by Drug Action Team area

Index of Organisations

1M/129/7